MOTIVATIONAL INTERVIEWING
WITH ADOLESCENTS AND YOUNG ADULTS

APPLICATIONS OF MOTIVATIONAL INTERVIEWING

Stephen Rollnick and William R. Miller, Series Editors

Since the publication of Miller and Rollnick's classic *Motivational Interviewing*, MI has become hugely popular as a tool for facilitating many different kinds of positive behavior change. This highly practical series demonstrates MI approaches for a range of applied contexts and with a variety of populations. Each accessible volume reviews the empirical evidence base and presents easy-to-implement strategies, illuminating concrete examples, and clear-cut guidance on integrating MI with other interventions.

Motivational Interviewing in the Treatment of Psychological Problems
*Hal Arkowitz, Henny A. Westra, William R. Miller,
and Stephen Rollnick, Editors*

**Motivational Interviewing in Health Care:
Helping Patients Change Behavior**
*Stephen Rollnick, William R. Miller,
and Christopher C. Butler*

Building Motivational Interviewing Skills: A Practitioner Workbook
David B. Rosengren

Motivational Interviewing with Adolescents and Young Adults
Sylvie Naar-King and Mariann Suarez

Motivational Interviewing with Adolescents and Young Adults

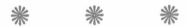

Sylvie Naar-King
Mariann Suarez

THE GUILFORD PRESS
New York   *London*

© 2011 The Guilford Press
A Division of Guilford Publications, Inc.
72 Spring Street, New York, NY 10012
www.guilford.com

Printed in the United States of America

This book is printed on acid-free paper.

Last digit is print number: 9   8   7   6   5   4

Library of Congress Cataloging-in-Publication Data
Naar-King, Sylvie.
    Motivational interviewing with adolescents and young adults / Sylvie Naar-
King, Mariann Suarez.
        p. cm. — (Applications of motivational interviewing)
    Includes bibliographical references and index.
    ISBN 978-1-60918-062-1 (hardcover)
    1. Motivational interviewing. 2. Teenagers. 3. Young adults. I. Suarez,
Mariann. II. Title.
    BF637.I5N293 2011
    158.'390835—dc22
                                                                        2010025132

*To the young people and families
who allowed us to share in their journey of change*

About the Authors

Sylvie Naar-King, PhD, is Associate Professor in the Department of Pediatrics and the Department of Psychiatry and Behavioral Neurosciences at Wayne State University. A pediatric psychologist, she conducts research on motivational and family therapy interventions for youth with HIV, asthma, diabetes, and obesity, and for adolescent risk reduction. Dr. Naar-King is a member of the Motivational Interviewing Network of Trainers (MINT) and is responsible for the MI training of medical residents at the Children's Hospital of Michigan.

Mariann Suarez, PhD, ABPP, is Head of Child Psychology and Assistant Professor in the Department of Psychiatry and Behavioral Medicine at the University of South Florida College of Medicine. She is a pediatric psychologist whose research focuses on the use of MI in the areas of substance misuse, child abuse and parenting, and the training of medical students and community practitioners. Dr. Suarez is a Diplomate in Cognitive and Behavioral Psychology of the American Board of Professional Psychology, a Fellow of the American Academy of Cognitive and Behavioral Psychology, and a member of MINT.

Contributing Authors

Ashley Austin, PhD, is Assistant Professor in the School of Social Work at Barry University. Her research interests focus on adolescent substance abuse, with a particular emphasis on interventions that strive to eliminate barriers to treatment for vulnerable subgroups of youth. Dr. Austin's publications are concentrated in the areas of adolescent substance abuse, motivationally based interventions, evidence-based practice, and racial/ethnic treatment disparities in treatment response and retention. Dr. Austin was a recipient of the 2008 National Institute on Drug Abuse Early Career Social Work Research Mentoring Initiative Award.

Elizabeth Barnett, MSW, is a doctoral student in Preventive Medicine at the University of Southern California. She is an active MI trainer and researcher. Her interests include adolescent substance use and obesity prevention interventions.

Nancy Barnett, PhD, is a clinical psychologist and Associate Professor (Research) in the Center for Alcohol and Addiction Studies in the Department of Community Health at Brown University. Her primary research areas are developing and testing brief interventions for substance use among adolescents and young adults, how change occurs following alcohol-related critical events, and the use of Internet-based and transdermal alcohol detection technologies for the assessment and treatment of alcohol use disorders.

Angela Bryan, PhD, is Professor and Director of the Health Psychology PhD Program in the Department of Psychology and a faculty member in the Center for Alcoholism, Substance Abuse, and Addictions at the University of New Mexico. Her research takes a transdisciplinary approach to the study of health and risk behavior, and the development of interventions to improve health behavior. She was the 2006 recipient of the American Psychological Association Distinguished Scientific Award for Early Career Contribution to Psychology in the area of Health Psychology.

Sue Channon, DClinPsych, is a clinical psychologist working in child health in a community pediatric setting. She has been involved in research developing the use of MI in working with teenagers with diabetes and, as a systemic practitioner, she has a particular interest in the application of MI in work with families.

Thomas H. Chun, MD, is Associate Professor in the Department of Emergency Medicine, Alpert Medical School, Brown University. His research interests include individual and family interventions for substance-using adolescents.

Elizabeth J. D'Amico, PhD, is Senior Behavioral Scientist at RAND Corporation and a licensed clinical psychologist. She is nationally recognized for her work developing, implementing, and evaluating alcohol and drug interventions for adolescents.

Jaimie Davis, RN, PhD, is Assistant Professor in the Department of Preventive Medicine, Keck School of Medicine, University of Southern California. Her research focuses on designing and disseminating nutrition, physical activity, and behavioral interventions to reduce obesity and related metabolic disorders in adolescents. She has a strong background in nutrition, physical activity, and body composition assessment in pediatric populations.

Deborah Ann Ellis, PhD, is Associate Professor in the Department of Pediatrics at Wayne State University. Her research interests focus on the reduction of health disparities in high-risk youth through behavioral interventions. She has significant interests in the areas of community-based family interventions for youth with HIV infection, asthma, and obesity.

Brett Engle, PhD, LCSW, is Assistant Professor at the Barry University School of Social Work. He is an active member of the Motivational Interviewing Network of Trainers. His research and practice interests include medical and community-based individual and group interventions for adolescent health risk behaviors.

Sarah W. Feldstein Ewing, PhD, is Assistant Professor of Translational Neuroscience at the Mind Research Network in Albuquerque, New Mexico. Her clinical and research interests focus on improving psychosocial interventions for health risk behaviors (including substance use, risky sexual behavior, and overeating) for adolescents and adults of all backgrounds. In addition to working on reducing health disparities in adolescent substance use interventions, Dr. Feldstein Ewing has been using translational approaches (including neuroimaging and genetics) to identify active ingredients of psychosocial interventions with the goal of improving intervention efficacy.

Nina Gobat, BSc, is an occupational therapist and doctoral student at the School of Medicine, Cardiff University, with clinical experience in general psychiatry and substance misuse. She is an active member of the Motivational Interviewing Network of Trainers and provides teaching and supervision to a range of health professionals. Her research and practice interests focus on communication, motivation, and behavior change.

Monique Green-Jones, MPH, is Research Assistant and Manager of the Horizons Project, a comprehensive continuum of care program for youth ages 13–24 at Wayne State University. She serves on the state HIV planning group and has experience in program and research management and evaluation and intervention implementation.

Lynn Hernandez, PhD, is Assistant Professor (Research) in the Center for Alcohol and Addiction Studies at Brown University. Her primary research interests focus on the development of culturally appropriate prevention and intervention programs for adolescents of diverse ethnic and racial backgrounds. She also has interest in examining the role that ethnocultural variables play in adolescents' substance use and other risk trajectories, and how these variables also influence adolescents' response to psychosocial treatments.

Kimberly Horn, EdD, MSW, is Robert C. Byrd Associate Professor of Community Medicine at West Virginia University. She is the Associate Center Director of Population Health Research at the Mary Babb Randolph Cancer Center and Co-Director of the WV Prevention Research Center. Dr. Horn is a nationally recognized expert in teen tobacco use and cessation. Most notably, she is the co-developer of the Not On Tobacco teen smoking cessation program. Other areas of expertise include intervention development and community-based participatory research.

Sarah Hunter, PhD, is a behavioral scientist at RAND Corporation and Professor at the Pardee RAND Graduate School. Her research interests stem from a desire to improve the quality of substance abuse prevention and treatment. Dr. Hunter has extensive experience in community participatory research and studying program implementation using both qualitative and quantitative methods.

Sebastian Kaplan, PhD, is a clinical psychologist and Assistant Professor in the Department of Psychiatry and Behavioral Medicine, Child and Adolescent Psychiatry Section, Wake Forest University School of Medicine. He is also a member of the Motivational Interviewing Network of Trainers, providing training in MI for mental health providers, health care practitioners, and school-based professionals. His clinical and research interests include the application of MI for adolescents and families.

Juline Koken, PhD, is an MI therapist, supervisor, trainer, and treatment fidelity expert. She has collaborated on research implementing MI to reduce risk behavior among youth both in the United States and internationally. She is currently Director of Research at the Center for Motivation and Change in New York City.

Carolina López, PhD, is a clinical psychologist for adolescents and Assistant Professor in the Faculty of Medicine at the University of Chile. She has been working with adolescents with eating disorders and their families since 1999.

Pam Macdonald, MSc, is currently working on her PhD at Kings College London, where she is part of a team looking at the effects of a DVD skills-based training project on caregiving. She also supports caregivers by coaching them using the principles of MI.

Lisa J. Merlo, PhD, is a licensed clinical psychologist and Assistant Professor of Psychiatry at the University of Florida College of Medicine. She is a member of the Motivational Interviewing Network of Trainers and specializes in clinical work with child/adolescent and pediatric patients. Dr. Merlo's research focuses primarily on psychosocial factors associated with compulsive and addictive behaviors.

Karen Chan Osilla, PhD, is a behavioral scientist at RAND Corporation. Her research interests include designing and evaluating brief interventions that use MI with at-risk teen and adult populations. She is currently involved in pilot studies evaluating in-person and Web-based brief interventions in employee assistance programs, driving under the influence programs, and teen courts.

Angulique Outlaw, PhD, is Assistant Professor in the Department of Pediatrics at Wayne State University School of Medicine. She is also Director of Prevention and Outreach Services for the Horizons Project of the Children's Hospital of Michigan, a comprehensive continuum-of-care program for HIV-infected and at-risk adolescents and young adults. Her research interests include prevention interventions, HIV risk behaviors, and retention in HIV care for youth.

Ken Resnicow, PhD, is Professor in the Department of Health Behavior and Health Education at the University of Michigan School of Public Health. His research interests include the design and evaluation of health promotion programs for special populations, particularly chronic disease prevention for African Americans; health communications; understanding the relationship between ethnicity and health behaviors; substance use prevention and harm reduction; and training health professionals to conduct MI interventions for obesity and other chronic diseases.

Sune Rubak, MD, PhD, is a consultant in the Department of Pediatrics at Skejby University Hospital and Associate Professor in Postgraduate Medical Education at the University of Aarhus. She has published several peer-reviewed papers on MI in international journals. Her main interest is in the development of MI theory and practice in the context of children and youth.

Holly Sindelar-Manning, PhD, is a clinical psychologist in the Children's Neurodevelopment Center at Hasbro Children's Hospital in Providence, Rhode Island. She treats and supports families of children and adolescents with developmental, behavioral, and social–emotional needs.

Anthony Spirito, PhD, is Professor of Psychiatry and Human Behavior, Alpert Medical School, Brown University. He has been conducting research on brief interventions for substance-abusing adolescents for the past 12 years.

Donna Spruijt-Metz, PhD, is Associate Professor in Preventive Medicine at the Keck School of Medicine, University of Southern California. She is an active member of the Motivational Interviewing Network of Trainers. Her research is in the field of pediatric obesity, with interests in the etiology, treatment, and prevention of childhood obesity, particularly in minority youth.

L. A. R. Stein, PhD, is Associate Professor in the Department of Psychology at the University of Rhode Island Social Sciences Research Center, Director of Research for the RI Training School, and Adjunct Faculty in Brown University's Department of Psychiatry and Human Behavior. She has an active program of study on behavioral interventions, including MI, for substance-using justice-involved persons. Her interests include MI as applied to adults, adolescents, and families; individual and group-based treatments; dissemination and implementation of treatment approaches to reduce risky behaviors; organizational change; and development of assessment tools.

Janet Treasure, PhD, is a Fellow of the Royal College of Psychiatrists, Royal College of Physicians, and the Academy of Eating Disorders. She heads the eating disorders services run by South London and Maudsley NHS Foundation Trust and has an academic appointment at Kings College London. As well as editing professional texts, she has written several self-help books for people with eating disorders and their caregivers.

Eric F. Wagner, PhD, is Director of Florida International University's Community Based Intervention Research Group and Professor in the University's Stempel College of Public Health and Social Work. He is an internationally recognized expert on brief interventions for teenage alcohol and drug users.

Denise Walker, PhD, is Research Assistant Professor in the School of Social Work at the University of Washington and Co-Director of the Innovative Programs Research Group. Her research focuses on the development and evaluation of interventions for marijuana, alcohol, substance abuse, and domestic violence.

Series Editors' Note

Motivational interviewing (MI) originated in the addictions field, in efforts to find constructive ways of responding to clients who were described as resistant, angry, defensive, and "in denial." Adolescents and young adults express these qualities routinely, with a flexibility that reminds us that they are perfectly normal reactions. It is therefore no surprise that, as MI spread into different fields, it found a home among practitioners working with children and young adults.

MI focuses on building constructive relationships with clients. The practical implication is a simple one, and it shines out of this book: Instead of labeling clients as resistant, try to see their ambivalence about changing as a challenge to your relationship with them, adjust your response, and the resistance will subside. Put another way, if a young person lies to his or her parents and not his or her best friend, the obvious conclusion is not that this young person is "a liar," but that one relationship is different from the other. How to use your privileged role as a helper to talk about meaningful change is one of the primary goals of MI.

This book is the only one of its kind to date—a practitioner's guide to how MI might look and feel in this area of new application. It's one thing to state that MI has a comfortable home in this area, quite another to assimilate and describe how everyday practice challenges might be overcome. Drs. Naar-King and Suarez, and their colleagues, have done an admirable job in bringing these challenges to life, and we thank them and The Guilford Press for contributing this volume to the expanding Applications of Motivational Interviewing series.

STEPHEN ROLLNICK
WILLIAM R. MILLER

Preface

Most of our work involves talking with young people, and if they have one thing in common, it is probably sensitivity to how they are spoken to. Yet the focus of so many interventions is on content, not process, on *what* to do but not *how* to do it. Motivational interviewing (MI) specifies how to guide people toward behavior change by paying very close attention to how we talk to them. What are the words we can say to increase the likelihood that young people will think about change? How can we encourage engagement instead of rebellion? And the words must come from a spirit of respect for the individual's capacity for change, a respect young people are often not afforded. Although many aspects of language are culturally specific, we have found the principles of MI and the developmental challenges of adolescence to be remarkably consistent across cultures.

In this book we have taken Miller and Rollnick's (1991) original presentation of MI, reflected on our own practice and that of others, absorbed the scientific evidence, and laid out how MI has been and might be used with young people. Inevitably we found that colleagues had applied MI in new and exciting contexts, which is why we decided to use contributed chapters in Part II of this volume.

Diverse applications of any method will result in innovation and adaptation that move away from the original statement of the method itself. This otherwise healthy process carries a risk that the method itself becomes too diffuse. We hope we have avoided this risk by staying true to the principles of MI, emphasizing that MI is essentially a conversation about change in which you strategically reinforce another's own motivation to change in the context of a respectful, empathic relationship. We hope you will dip into and out of this book as you learn how to use core skills and attend to the spirit and the language that produce less frustrating and more satisfying interactions with young people.

Acknowledgments

We would like to thank our family, friends, mentors, and work colleagues who helped us create the time and space to write this book. We would like to thank members of the Motivational Interviewing Network of Trainers for their willingness to ponder our questions. While we cannot possibly name all the people who helped and inspired us, we wanted to particularly thank those who reviewed earlier versions of this text. Steven Rollnick has been so affirming and supportive and pushed us to write beyond the confines of academia. William R. Miller is always open to new ideas and specifically encouraged us to "keep thinking." Katie Brogan, Nikki Cockern, Raymond Courtney, Robert Kender, and Lisa Merlo all read chapters and gave invaluable feedback from different perspectives. Finally, thank you, Bill, Steve, and Guilford's Senior Editor Jim Nageotte for believing in us.

Contents

PART III. CHOOSING YOUR OWN PATH

PART I

✳ ✳ ✳

THE GUIDE

CHAPTER 1

❋　　❋　　❋　　❋

Introduction

Why Motivational Interviewing with Adolescents and Young Adults?

They mustn't know my despair, I can't let them see the wounds which they have caused, I couldn't bear their sympathy and their kind-hearted jokes, it would only make me want to scream all the more. If I talk, everyone thinks I'm showing off; when I'm silent they think I'm ridiculous; rude if I answer, sly if I get a good idea, lazy if I'm tired, selfish if I eat a mouthful more than I should, stupid, cowardly, crafty, etc. etc.
—ANNE FRANK, *The Diary of Anne Frank*

If you work with adolescents and young adults, you are well aware that young people present with unique challenges and opportunities. Rates of risk behaviors, such as unprotected sex and substance use peak in adolescence and emerging adulthood (Park, Mulye, Adams, Brindis, & Irwin, 2006). Poor health behaviors such as sedentary activity and poor self-management of medical conditions set the stage for lifelong health problems. Conflict with parents and pressure from peers contribute additional stress. These life challenges often result in young people who feel misunderstood in a society that pathologizes them. "I would there were no age between ten and three-and-twenty, or that youth would sleep out the rest; for there is nothing in the between but getting wenches with child, wronging the ancientry, stealing, fighting" (William Shakespeare, *The Winter's Tale*, Act III, Scene 3). If you can break through the sense of alienation often experienced by young clients, you have a great advantage. Not only can you make a genuine connection, but also you have an opportunity to maximize the young person's potential during a period of tremendous growth and development. Chapter 2 reviews adolescent development in further detail.

3

If you work with adolescents and young adults, you are faced with a complicated task. With each client, you are challenged to balance many developmental and contextual factors, while simultaneously following the client's own agenda. Consider the example of Jenny, a 15-year-old female referred for obesity treatment and decide how you might proceed:

> Since childhood, Jenny has struggled with weight, currently exceeding 60 pounds over a healthy body mass index. She has always been an above-average student, but this past year has become avoidant of school and her grades are dropping. She "jokes" about how others tease her, yet you sense a depressed mood. When discussing treatment options, she says she's "tried it all," and confides she will "do whatever *you* want *me* to do," but doesn't see much hope for change. She also notes that there are certain foods she will not give up, and she does not see herself ever going to a gym. Her parents are divorced. Her mother is the primary caregiver, though she visits her father on the weekends. Both Jenny and her mother complain that the father stocks the house with junk food and sits around and watches TV all day. Her mother also struggles with obesity and does not think Jenny is "that fat." Coming to you is fine if that's what she wants to do, but she has a busy schedule with a full-time job and cannot bring her to many appointments.

Although this scenario may present several options for empirically supported interventions (e.g., self-monitoring of food intake, cognitive-behavioral treatment of depression, behavior plans for exercise), an unmotivated adolescent can block any suggestion you may offer—stifling even the most seamless of recommendations! Even when the focus of treatment is with the parent (e.g., to increase monitoring, to administer rewards and consequences), interventions are much more difficult to implement when the adolescent is unwilling to engage. Most treatments for adolescents and young adults are developed for patients who are ready to change, and you may often feel frustrated when the young person does not follow your recommendations. Perhaps this is why Trepper (1991) described working with adolescents as an "adversarial sport" in which you rarely end up on the winning team. However, those of you who have chosen to work with adolescents know that their energy, intensity, and capacity for change make the challenges worthwhile, and motivational interviewing can help turn these challenges into opportunities.

If you have experienced this frustration and joy when working with young people, this book is for you. It is our hope to provide you with a guide for having a productive conversation about behavior change with adolescents and young adults using the spirit and skills of motivational interviewing (MI). Although MI is a widely effective behavior change method specified in the early 1980s with adults, it has been slower to permeate into pediatric and family practice. In the past decade, however, research on MI with young people has blossomed. With this book, it is our hope to meet the need practitioners have voiced for an MI resource tailored to the unique developmental context of adolescence and young adulthood. While we are all clinical psychologists by training, we believe the spirit and skills presented in this book are applicable to a variety of practitioners and settings.

WHAT IS MI?

MI is a collaborative, person-centered form of guiding to elicit and strengthen motivation for change (Miller & Rollnick, 2009). MI should not be viewed as a technique, trick, or something to be done to people to make them change. Rather, it is a gentle, respectful method for communicating with others about their difficulties with change and the possibilities to engage in different, healthier behaviors that are in accord with their own goals and values to maximize human potential.

What MI Is Not

While MI is a learnable and effective method for enhancing motivation for healthy behavior change, the process for acquiring proficiency in these skills requires effort and practice. Miller and Rollnick (2009) discussed several common misunderstandings practitioners frequently encounter when learning MI. Understanding what MI is not will help you understand what MI is!

MI Is Not Based on a Theory or School of Psychotherapy

MI emerged by specifying practitioner behaviors associated with behavior change in treatment session recordings. A common misconception, even for those well versed in MI, is that MI is based on a specific theory, often, the transtheoretical model of change (TTM; Prochaska & DiClemente, 1984), also known as the stages-of-change model. The TTM was developed parallel with MI and helped to open the door to appreciating the need for interventions for those who are not fully ready to change. Another theory of motivation consistent with an MI approach, self-determination theory (Deci & Ryan, 1985), explains the continuum from extrinsic to intrinsic motivation and is utilized in the next chapter to help illustrate the spirit of MI. Social cognitive theories such as the information–motivation–behavior skills model (Fisher, Fisher, & Harman, 2003) have also been described as underlying MI-based interventions. Clearly, MI may be consistent with many theories, but in truth MI is an example of grounded theory. That is, the method emerged from the data (session recordings), and only now is a theory beginning to be explicated (Miller & Rose, 2009).

> MI is not based in a specific school of psychotherapy, nor is it meant to be a treatment for all problems and conditions.

Similarly, MI is not based in a specific school of psychotherapy, nor is it meant to be a treatment for all problems and conditions. While MI makes use of client-centered counseling skills (Rogers, 1959), it includes more goal-oriented components. You will not follow the young person wherever he or she wants to go, but rather you will guide him or her into maximizing potential. In this way, the client-centered approach is a necessary but not sufficient condition. Yet, MI is also not a directive approach, as in cognitive-behavioral treatment. Cognitive-behavioral treatments offer young patients something they don't have, such as a behavioral skill or a cognitive coping strategy. MI is about eliciting internal motivation and strengths when ambivalence is impeding behavior change. Skills and strategies may then be offered when the young person is ready to make change.

MI Is Not a Bag of Tricks and Techniques

A major difference between MI and other approaches is that it is not manualized and should not be viewed as a cookbook, bag of tricks, or set of techniques that you can apply *to* young persons or families. The MI method emphasizes empathy, honesty, and collaboration. You respect the young person as being the expert of him- or herself and as possessing the mechanisms and internal resources to make a change (i.e., personal values, motivations, abilities, skills) with or without your advice. Moreover, MI is a style or spirit without which the techniques fall flat. This style is defined further in the next chapter, and this spirit is the first task in learning MI. Some MI-based interventions have focused on specific techniques, such as the decisional balance exercise (examining the pros and cons of behavior change) or use of assessment feedback (objective review of assessment tools to heighten awareness of the need for behavior change). Although these strategies may be included in MI (see Chapters 5 and 6), they do not define it.

MI Is Not Easy to Learn

Learning MI is similar to an athletic person learning a new sport. You already have a repertoire of skills as a foundation, but becoming proficient in MI requires more than a review of a text, or attendance at a 2-day workshop (Miller & Mount, 2001; Miller, Yahne, Moyers, Martinez, & Pirritano, 2004). MI proficiency involves a process of learning, practicing, and receiving feedback, both from others in the field and from young people in your clinical encounters (see Part III).

WHAT'S THE EVIDENCE?

MI was developed as a brief intervention for problem drinkers and debuted in a 1983 paper published by William R. Miller in *Behavioural Psychotherapy* (Miller, 1983). The fundamental concepts targeted in this initial intervention—namely, motivation and the obstacles it poses for change—were later elaborated in 1991 by William R. Miller and Stephen Rollnick in the seminal text, *Motivational Interviewing: Preparing People for Change*. A second revised edition of the text was published in 2002. A third edition is in press. Subsequent to these publications, an array of MI-based interventions for adults began to emerge, primarily targeting substance use, but also focusing on mental health problems and health behaviors in adults (Hettema, Steele, & Miller, 2005).

In recent years, research investigating the effects of MI with younger populations has emerged. Clinical outcome studies have shown that MI has positive effects in substance-using adolescents and young adults. Evidence is emerging to support the efficacy of MI for other behaviors as well, such as smoking, sexual risk, eating disorders and obesity, chronic illness management, and externalizing and internalizing behavior problems. The chapters at the end of the book describe interventions for these specific problems and provide references for the evidence base.

HOW IS THIS GUIDE ORGANIZED?

If you are wishing you remembered the developmental information you may have received over the course of your education, Chapter 2 reviews the development of adolescence and young adulthood in more detail. We then move on to presenting MI as a pyramid with MI spirit at the foundation and commitment to change at the top.

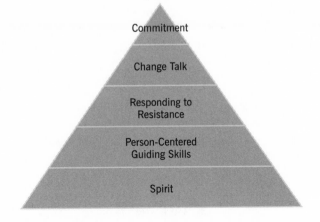

Chapter 3 focuses on understanding the spirit of motivational interviewing, for mastering skills without the spirit is like learning the words of a song without hearing the music. Chapter 4 concentrates on person-centered guiding skills, core micro-skills used not only for the patient-centered components of developing rapport and expressing empathy, but also for the more goal-oriented aspects of MI. Chapter 5 presents skills that will help you respond to resistance, skills we believe are worth mastering early because resistance and ambivalence are likely to emerge at the onset of treatment with young people. Chapter 6 focuses on self-motivating statements (change talk)—how to recognize these statements, how to verbally reinforce them to increase commitment, and how to elicit them if they do not occur spontaneously when you are exploring the young person's point of view. Chapter 7 addresses how to consolidate commitment and how to develop change plans necessary for actual behavior change. Finally, in Chapter 8, we discuss how to integrate MI with other interventions. In the second section of the book, contributors specializing in specific youth behaviors describe MI interventions for commonly encountered issues. The text concludes with a summary of ethical issues and suggestions for future training.

SUMMARY

Young people present with both challenges and opportunities, and we invite you to begin your own journey of learning the MI method to promote behavior change in this population. While the following chapters offer a useful guide, the path each of us will take in incorporating these principles and skills into daily practice will vary. Some are drawn to the person-centered components of MI and struggle with the more goal-oriented strategies. Others move to goal attainment and behavior change planning too quickly and struggle to maintain a person-centered stance. Akin to the young person's journey of change, your journey to learn MI will include many challenges and opportunities. In the following chapters, we hope to guide you to incorporate MI in your clinical practice and encourage you to continue the journey of change beyond this book.

SUMMARY: MAJOR ASPECTS OF MI

What is MI?	A collaborative, person-centered form of guiding to elicit and strengthen motivation for change
What is MI not?	1. Theory laden 2. A trick to make people do what you want 3. A technique

	4. A decisional balance 5. Assessment feedback 6. A subclass of cognitive-behavioral therapy 7. The same as client-centered counseling 8. Easy to learn 9. What you are already doing because you recognize it 10. A panacea
How do I know when to use MI?	When the young person expresses low motivation, hesitancy to engage in treatment, or difficulty in changing behavior.
How do I know when not to use MI?	With the small percentage of young persons who are motivated and sufficiently ready to change.
What is the evidence base?	• Blossoming in all areas including health, mental health, and judicial. • A few studies with ages 11, most on ages 13 and older.
How is MI different with young persons and families?	• The unique developmental context of adolescence and emerging adulthood suggests that the behavior change journey will differ from that of adults. • Prevents myths of developmental uniformity (i.e., they're all the same) and continuity (i.e., adult therapies can be used the same with young persons) from negatively impacting your intervention.

What are the major developmental factors to consider when using MI?	• Biological
	• Cognitive
	• Social
	  o Identity
	  o Autonomy
	  o Relationships with family and peers

What are the eight tasks for learning MI?	1. The spirit of MI 2. Person-centered guiding skills 3. Rolling with resistance 4. Recognizing and reinforcing change talk 5. Eliciting change talk 6. Developing a change plan 7. Consolidating commitments 8. Integrating MI with other treatments
What is the MI invitation?	An invitation to begin your own journey to learn MI. Caution: *You* may change.

✳ ✳ ✳ ✳

Adolescence and Emerging Adulthood

A Brief Review of Development

> Adolescents are not monsters. They are just people trying
> to learn how to make it among the adults in the world,
> who are probably not so sure themselves.
> —Virginia Satir

A Brief Review of Cognitive Development

MI requires the young person to take responsibility and be an active part of the decision to change (or not). You will explore the young person's thoughts about the target behavior as well as expectations about the future possibilities and consequences of taking action. An understanding of how the young person's cognitive processes differ from those of adults will help you to have these conversations. We next review two major approaches to cognitive development: the Piagetian approach and the information-processing approach.

Formal Operations

Piaget (1967, 1971, 1972) developed a comprehensive stage theory of cognitive development emphasizing the broad patterns and qualitative changes occurring during this period. Of relevance to the application of MI is the final stage of cognitive development beginning during early adolescence (ages 11–12 years), the formal operational stage. During this period, the cognitive process of reasoning and formal thinking patterns radically changes and develops. The further along the young person is in this stage, the more likely you will be able to have conversations about ambivalence and possible plans for change. Adolescents with less cognitively developed resources will require that you tailor your discussions to short-term and concrete changes. Older adolescents and/or those with more developed cognitive processes may benefit from conversations targeting longer-term goals and values.

> Adolescents with less cognitively developed resources will require that you tailor your discussions to short-term and concrete changes. Older adolescents and/or those with more developed cognitive processes may benefit from conversations targeting longer-term goals and values.

Information Processing

The information-processing approach examines the young person's perception, attention, retrieval, and manipulation of information (Siegler, 1995). Two information-processing steps are particularly relevant for MI with young people.

Interpretation

Past experiences help to guide accurate judgment and analysis of facts. Young people, however, often lack the necessary life experiences to facilitate accurate judgments. Thus, they are more susceptible to interpretational biases (Rice & Dolgin, 2008). For example, a young person making his or her initial sexual debut may forgo the use of protection from lack of experience and belief that this behavior will not result in unwanted consequences, such as a sexually transmitted disease or pregnancy.

Higher-Order Thought Processes

Interestingly, young people often rely on negative information and use disconfirming evidence. Thus, they seek to negate rather than affirm, using elimination strategies rather than confirmation strategies in their thinking (Foltz, Overton, & Ricco, 1995; Mueller, Sokol, & Overton, 1999; Rice & Dolgin, 2008). For example, young persons who are considering quitting smoking may well understand the health risks involved with smoking, yet believe there is no risk due to their young age and potential to stop at any time they choose.

A Brief Review
of Social and Emotional Development

Identity and role formulation has been described as one of the most important tasks of the young person's development (Baumeister, 1991; Cole et al., 2001; Rice & Dolgin, 2008). During this transitional period, the young person's self-concept stabilizes (Arnett, 2004; Cole et al., 2001), and experimentation with different behaviors and values increases (Rice & Dolgin, 2008). Deciding to make long-term changes at this point in the developmental period can be hard for young people, as they are trying on new roles that tend to be more temporary, rather than stable across time. However, knowledge of the central issues surrounding social role development provides you the opportunity to more efficiently partner with the young person, while concurrently respecting their need to explore and establish personal values and goals.

> Deciding to make long-term changes at this point in the developmental period can be hard for young people, as they are trying on new roles that tend to be more temporary, rather than stable across time.

Identity and Adolescence

Erickson (1950, 1968, 1982) defined eight stages of psychosocial personality development. Adolescence is characterized by the fifth stage, identity versus diffusion. During this stage, the goal of establishing a personal identity is achieved by evaluating one's own personal positive and negative qualities to help clarify one's self-concept, and determine the type of adult one wants to become in the future (Rice & Dolgin, 2008). Identity formation occurs through multiple role explorations and commitments to various life issues (i.e., occupational, academic, religious, social, sexual, and political) (Holmbeck, O'Mahar, Abad, Colder, & Updegrove, 2006). Understanding the purpose of multiple role explorations in forming identity will help you express accurate empathy.

Identity and Emerging Adulthood

In the past half decade, historical societal and economic changes have created new demands and challenges for young people, particularly those in the 18- to 25-year-old range, making it a distinct period separate from adolescence and young adulthood, termed "emerging adulthood" (Arnett, 2004). During this period, emerging adults experience new life roles. Recent research by Arnett (2004) has shown that the length of time for young persons to actually create an identity has increased to the mid- to late 20s. You should be aware that emerging adulthood in Western culture is still a time of shifting identities. There is a continued risk of experimentation with unhealthy behaviors, perhaps even an increased risk as the young person is no longer a minor and is faced with two additional life challenges: increased adult responsibilities and decreased familial support (Arnett, 2004).

Autonomy

A core element in the journey to adulthood involves the attainment of autonomy (Rice & Dolgin, 2008). During this time, young people establish their uniqueness from others, and new interests, values, goals, and world-views divergent from close others may emerge (Rice & Dolgin, 2008). A normal developmental process, autonomy has been described as having two components: emotional and behavioral autonomy. Emotional autonomy refers to becoming free of childish emotional dependence on adults (Rice & Dolgin, 2008). Largely dependent on parental behavior, parents can foster overdependence on the developing young person, as well as provide the opposite, a lack of guidance and support, with a balance of both being the most preferred course of action (Rice & Dolgin, 2008). Behavioral autonomy refers to the adolescents becoming skilled in their own self-governing behavior and independent enough to make decisions on their own accord, without depending on others for consultation or advice (Holmbeck et al., 2006; Rice & Dolgin, 2008). While discussed in greater detail in Chapter 3, autonomy in decision making and the taking of responsibility for actions in MI serves as a fundamental component of the method (Miller & Rollnick, 2002). These issues become an especially important part of intervention with adolescents and family members, as young persons are faced with the developmental conundrum of exploring alternative behaviors and roles that smack of adultlike decisions, while being confined by parental and societal regulations.

Family and Peers

The period of adolescence has gotten a bad rap, with public perceptions of young persons as "rude and irresponsible" being the norm (Holmbeck et al., 2006; Public Agenda, 1999). Moreover, the belief that this period is a time to sever ties with parents or develop significant mental health disorders pervades clinical lore (Collins & Laursen, 1992). However, research provides us with a more optimistic analysis of this period: It can be a time of role transformations in family relationships and increasing personal responsibility and decision-making authority (Holmbeck, 1996; Steinberg, 1990). Any increases in conflict and negative emotions toward family members are considered a normal part of development, with disagreements serving an adaptive function of facilitating the young person's negotiation in decision making and autonomy within the family unit (Holmbeck, 1996).

Similar to family relationships, peers serve an important function during the young person's development (Holmbeck et al., 2006; Parker & Asher, 1987; Rice & Dolgin, 2008; Steinberg, 2005). During this stage, friendships become both a primary and a stressful part of the young person's life. Social acceptance by peers tends to foster overall well-being, while rejection often leads to engagement in more problematic behaviors (i.e., delinquency, drug abuse, and depression) (Merten, 1996).

Young people mastering the tasks of autonomous decision making typically rely on the feedback of close others, especially peers. Your understanding of the young person's perceptions of these relationships can inform change talk discussions. For example, a young person may perceive drinking alcohol with peers as a positively rewarding experience, yet experience conflict with parents when engaging in these activities. Dependent on the nature of the relationship with parents and peers, the topics you raise during an MI encounter can differ. For example, if the teenager views parental approval as something of value and important, discussing the negative consequences received at home may be an appropriate focus to decrease ambivalence about drinking alcohol. However, if peer relationships are more valued than parental approval, conversations about family may increase ambivalence to consider change and resistant behaviors. Thus, incorporating family and peer relationship issues can provide you a window to explore how the young person perceives and relates to others, the value of relationships in their life, and access to integrating socially relevant topics central to change.

Emotional stress typically arises in the face of conflict with parents or peers. With young persons, emotions (and hormones) are often in a state of flux. Who among us can't recall the pangs of being a young person and experiencing some intense emotion, be it fear, anger, or sadness, over what now seems but a moment in the process of our development? It is important for you to recognize that cognitive processes may sometimes be compromised when the young person displays a heightened emotional state. During these times, your decision of how to intervene in an MI-consistent manner (i.e., taking only a supportive stance and eliciting a discussion about behavioral change at a later point) may require your clinical judgment. The emotional waves that often ride the tide of the young person's cognitive and decision-making abilities are often present, and your surfing skills, even when the emotional tides are high, can serve you in continuing to help the young person swim to his or her destination.

SUMMARY

Adolescence and emerging adulthood is defined as the transitional developmental period between childhood and adulthood, extending from ages 12 to the 20s. After infancy, it is the period of the greatest biological, psychological and social role changes (Arnett, 2004; Rice & Dolgin, 2008). The constant flux of change experienced during this period provides a prime opportunity to intervene and positively alter the trajectory of unhealthy behaviors and poor outcomes (Holmbeck et al., 2006). MI is different with young people because the normal developmental processes of adolescence regularly (and sometimes unpredictably!) affect the young person's motivations, decisions, and goals. An understanding of the cognitive and social emotional developmental processes described in this chapter will improve your ability to have conversations with young people to promote health behavior change.

SUMMARY: DEVELOPMENT AND MI IMPLICATIONS

Development	Implications for MI
Cognitive Development	
Formal operations	Consider implications for discussions of long-term goals and abstract values.
Information processing	May misinterpret consequences of behaviors and actively seek disconfirming evidence.
Social and Emotional Development	
Identity formation	Allow exploration of self-concept, empathize with ambivalence, and be tolerant of shifts in perspective.
Autonomy	Understand that opposition to authority is a normal developmental process.
Family	Help family members to reframe adolescent rebellion as normal process of identity formation.
Peers	Explore values and stresses associated with peers as possible pros and cons of behavior change.
Emotional lability	Be careful of making plans for change during period of intense emotion.

✳   ✳   ✳   ✳

The Spirit
of Motivational Interviewing

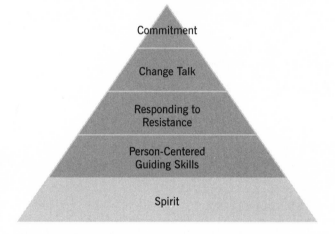

The word that allows yes, the word that makes no possible. The word that puts the free in freedom and takes the obligation out of love. The word that throws a window open after the final door is closed. The word upon which all adventure, all exhilaration, all meaning, all honor depends. The word that fires evolution's motor of mud. The word that the cocoon whispers to the caterpillar. The word that molecules recite before bonding. The word that separates that which is dead from that which is living. The word no mirror can turn around. *CHOICE.*
—TOM ROBBINS, *Still Life with Woodpecker*

MI is not a list of techniques, but rather a method or a style of interacting with patients. As such, the foundation of MI is its spirit. Miller (2008) has suggested that learning the techniques without the spirit is like learning the words to a song without the music. When learning a new song, you typically learn the tune first and then memorize the words. If you can hum the tune, then you are already halfway there. MI spirit is described by three themes. Miller and Rollnick use mnemonic devices throughout their original text to aid in the recollection of key components of MI. In keeping with this tradition, we present the themes as ACE—autonomy, collaboration, and evocation—and demonstrate how these themes are relevant to working with young people.

MI THEMES:
AUTONOMY, COLLABORATION, AND EVOCATION (ACE)

Autonomy

The development of autonomy is one of the key tasks of adolescence, and this independence of thoughts, feelings, and decisions is a basic human need (Deci & Ryan, 1985). If you inadvertently counter this need by pressuring the young person to change or by problem solving prematurely, you will experience the young person pushing away strongly. You have then elicited resistance instead of change. MI takes the stance that one person cannot *make* another person change. If we could, our jobs would be much easier, though possibly unethical. You might coerce a temporary behavior change with an incentive or punishment, but lasting change requires an internal process.

> If you inadvertently counter this need by pressuring the young person to change or by problem solving prematurely, you will experience the young person pushing away strongly. You have then elicited resistance instead of change.

Your job is not to take responsibility for change, but rather to support and guide while seeking to elicit the young person's own ideas for change even within a constrained environment (e.g., "your parents say you have certain chores to complete, but perhaps you can decide the best time of day to complete them"). Thus, you can provide an environment of "supportive autonomy" by eliciting the young person's perspectives, by providing information and a menu of options, and by emphasizing personal choice and responsibility (Williams, 2002).

Of course, when working with adolescents, you will likely need to be responsive to the constraints that authority figures pose (e.g., curfew), and you may in fact need to encourage such structure (e.g., parental monitoring). However, it is still possible to be supportive of autonomy within these limits by emphasizing personal choice. For example, "You have a choice to discuss the rules with your parents and see if there is room to compromise, or you can decide to break the rules and deal with your parents' reaction."

Collaboration

The MI spirit is collaborative—a partnership between you and the young person. This is in contrast to prescriptive approaches in which you are the expert handing down wisdom. While you will often need to collaborate with parents regarding goals, behavior change will not occur in the absence of a partnership with the youth. You may also experience a professional conundrum during this process, in which you are caught between the goals of authority figures and the goals of the young person. Of course, this is parallel to the pressure that the young person feels. The challenge is to guide the young person toward setting goals that will satisfy the need for autonomy *and* at the same time address the pressure to get along with authority figures.

Rollnick, Miller, and Butler (2008) expand on this guiding style. A guide helps people find their way safely and solve situations for themselves. Similar to a parent on the playground, there should be a balance of helping, supporting, and avoiding harm, while simultaneously allowing the child to experiment and problem-solve for him- or herself. Thus, collaboration involves a joint process, not merely serving the young person's impulses and desires, nor only satisfying your agenda. You must be honest (with yourself and the young person) about your role in promoting both autonomous decision making *and* positive behavior change in order to maximize the young person's potential. For example, a prescriptive approach to substance abuse treatment may insist on abstinence as the only solution, but a collaborative approach may consider a harm-reduction goal consistent with the young person's desire for change. However, as a guide it may be appropriate to offer information about the success of abstinence approaches when the young person is ready to hear it.

In the case of Jenny described in Chapter 1, a prescriptive approach might delineate calorie restrictions or engage the parents in setting limits around access to food. However, both of these strategies will be more likely to fail without collaboration of the young person. Alternatively, these interventions are more likely to succeed if, in conversation with the practitioner, Jenny determines that she is committed to losing weight by cutting calories and that her parents could help her by not purchasing chips and soda.

Evocation

In MI, you evoke and elicit reasons for and concerns about change, rather than imparting unsolicited advice. Thus, evocation may run counter to the natural instinct to "help" the young person by correcting what you construe as flawed reasoning or poor decision making. Miller and Rollnick (2002) describe this phenomenon as the *righting reflex*, the human tendency to correct things that are perceived as wrong. This tendency often translates into premature problem solving and advice giving, which prevents young people from being actively involved in the process, and actually places them in a passive role. This righting reflex stifles autonomy and can engender rebellion by the young person.

In Jenny's case, you may feel strongly pulled to correct misinformation about what it takes to lose weight (e.g., I can eat whatever I want as long as I exercise) without first understanding Jenny's thoughts and feelings about weight loss and other areas of her life. This can evoke resistance instead of motivation. Instead, you want to have Jenny argue for change and ask for information.

Evoking implies an active process that takes MI beyond client-centered counseling and into a goal-oriented intervention method. MI seeks to evoke intrinsic motivation—the engagement in behaviors for personal interest as opposed to external consequences. Although some behaviors will never be truly intrinsically motivated because they are not pleasurable (e.g., restricting sweets, taking insulin), the young person may still internalize motivation to engage in these behaviors by transforming external demands into personal values or goals. In many ways, this is the goal of the motivational interview. You will learn to do this by eliciting verbalizations about change so that the young person argues for change instead of you doing it for them.

> Although some behaviors will never be truly intrinsically motivated because they are not pleasurable (e.g., restricting sweets, taking insulin), the young person may still internalize motivation to engage in these behaviors by transforming external demands into personal values or goals. In many ways, this is the goal of the motivational interview.

TRANSLATING SPIRIT INTO PRACTICE

The ACE themes pertain to therapeutic stance, whereas four MI principles begin to demonstrate what you will actually do in an encounter with a young person: *express empathy, develop discrepancy, roll with resistance,* and *support self-efficacy.* Later chapters will address how to put these principles into practice.

Express Empathy

Adolescence is a time when young persons are separating from their parents, when relating to others is based more on personal ideas and decisions than on those of family members or authority figures. It is common for the young person to experience a lack of acceptance and understanding from adults, and communication with parents can deteriorate. Adolescents, particularly younger adolescents, may feel loved only conditionally, depending on their behavior and compliance with external demands. However, adolescents, like all of us, want someone to understand, listen, and believe they have something worthwhile to say (Rice & Dolgin, 2008). Thus, your display of empathy and acceptance is especially critical during MI encounters.

The concept of empathy has long been considered a key component in many different types of psychotherapy, both for the development of therapeutic alliance and for its therapeutic effect as an intervention to relieve personal distress. When you provide a secure and caring interpersonal context, you enhance the development of intrinsic motivation. For example, intrinsic motivation is lower in children who experience their teachers as cold and uncaring (Deci & Ryan, 1985). MI specifies ways to express empathy even within the confines of limited communication from the young person.

Develop Discrepancy

Behavior change is more likely to occur when the new behavior is identified as being consistent with the young person's own values and goals. When a client simply accepts the external demands and rules of others but does not believe in them, behavior change may occur as a result of threats, guilt, or shame. However, behavior change due to external forces is less stable and more inconsistent over time than change due to internal forces. Thus, you can promote behavior change by evoking, reflecting, and even magnifying the discrepancy between the young person's values and goals and their current status quo behaviors. Developing these discrepancies may compel the young person to consider and possibly change the status quo behaviors to coalesce with his or her own values. For example, for a young person who highly values personal independence, a discussion focusing on how drug use increases dependence (on the drug, on the dealer, on others for financial resources) may subsequently increase intrinsic motivation to avoid drugs.

In developing discrepancy, it is critical that you focus on the young person's behavior and values, not *your* values or social norms. The patient's values and goals may be external (e.g., having a girlfriend), short term (e.g., wanting to go to a party on Friday night), or unrealistic (e.g., wanting to be a rap star), but all values and goals may be utilized to promote motivation for change. For example, Jenny may be motivated to lose weight merely to look good to others and not for the sake of her own health. If you do not agree with the value (e.g., losing weight for appearance rather than health), it can be tempting to try to convince the person, "you know that losing weight is also really important for your health." However, this may result in the young person arguing against your advice. Instead, by curbing your value judgments and using the young person's own values to develop discrepancy (e.g., "I will begin exercising so that I can fit into this dress"), behavior change is more likely to occur (see Chapter 6).

Roll with Resistance

In MI, resistance is considered an interpersonal process and is met with clarification of the young person's point of view instead of correction or interpretation. Resistance has historically been considered a negative patient state or even trait. More recently, resistance in psychotherapy has been reconceptualized as an interpersonal process affected by both client and practitioner variables (Engle & Arkowitz, 2006; Freeman & McCloskey, 2001). Humans have a tendency to experience negative feelings (i.e., psychological reactance) when they perceive that their personal freedoms are limited or controlled (Brehm, 1966). In adolescents, these negative feelings may manifest in outright rebellion. Not surprisingly given the young person's focus on autonomy, psychological reactance has been shown to occur more frequently during adolescence and young adulthood (Hong, Giannakopoulos, Laing, & Williams, 1994) and may be especially likely when the young person has not come to treatment of his or her own accord.

When you sense resistance in the relationship or when you hear statements against change or in favor of the status quo (later referred to as "sustain talk," which is the opposite of "change talk"), we suggest the strategy of stop, drop, and roll. First, "stop" refers to pausing and considering the situation. Some questions you might ask yourself are: Is the young person focusing on why he or she should not change? Is he or she blaming others instead of focusing on taking responsibility? If so, you should next "drop" your current approach and try something different. Were you arguing for reasons to change? Drop it! Was the young person disagreeing with you about reasons not to change? Drop it! Next, you may need to "roll" with resistance, as this is critical to reducing further psychological reactance and sustain talk. Your goal in "rolling" with resistance is to not argue for change, but rather to express an understanding of the young person's point of view while emphasizing personal choice. The next chapter describes specific reflective listening skills that help you express this understanding to your young clients.

Support Self-Efficacy

Miller and Rollnick (2002) note that actual behavior change occurs in a client when he or she deems the behavior important *and* when he or she feels able to make the change. Young people often perceive themselves as falling short of the expectations of authority figures. When you take a stance of hope and optimism for successful behavior change and express an honest belief in the young person's ability, the young person is likely to feel more competent and therefore behavior change is more likely to occur. For example, an adolescent may acknowledge that marijuana use is a problem, but will not set a goal for abstinence or reduction of use without believing in a chance for success. This concept, referred to as self-efficacy, is the belief in one's ability to be competent in specific situations (e.g. "I can avoid alcohol during the week") and in specific tasks (e.g., "I can administer my insulin though I am struggling more with testing blood sugars." Your role as a guide is to help the young person find inner strength to build confidence for behavior change (see the sections "Affirmations" in Chapter 4 and "Questions about Personal Strengths" in Chapter 6).

DIFFERENCES BETWEEN MI AND OTHER APPROACHES

Now that you have a sense of MI spirit, you likely have begun to notice the differences between MI and other approaches. MI differs from more confrontational approaches in that the focus is on the individual's reasons for change instead of the pressure from external forces. However, MI also differs from nondirective approaches in that you are not simply following the person anywhere she wants to go, but rather are guiding her toward behavior change. Table 3.1 demonstrates differences between MI and other approaches to treatment.

TABLE 3.1 MI Compared to Other Approaches

Other approaches	MI: Person-centered *and* goal-oriented
Directive-only approaches	
You view the young person's acceptance of a diagnosis as essential for change.	You see that change can occur without the young person's acceptance of a "problem."
You emphasize your knowledge.	You emphasize the young person's personal choice and responsibility.
You see resistance as "denial"— something that must be confronted.	You see resistance as an interpersonal process influenced by your behavior.
You respond to resistance with interpretation or correction.	You respond to resistance with reflection to clarify the young person's viewpoint.
Nondirective approaches	
The young person determines the content and direction of the interaction.	You systematically guide toward motivation for change.
You avoid injecting advice and feedback.	You offer advice and feedback where appropriate and with permission.
You use empathic reflection unconditionally.	You use empathic reflection selectively to build motivation for change.

DEMONSTRATING SPIRIT IN THE INITIAL ENCOUNTER

Opening Statement

The first statement you offer to the young person should encompass the MI spirit. The key is to convey the idea that you will support the young person's desired changes (guiding), rather than direct which changes should be made. For example, in setting the stage for the encounter, you might say: "Our time today may be different than with other people who have talked to you. I am not here to tell you what to change or how to change, but rather to find out what is going on in your life and help you make the changes that you decide to make." With this type of opening statement, you can more effectively align with the young person and possibly be perceived as someone who is distinct from other authority figures in his or her life. Like adults who have been court-ordered to receive treatment, young people are typically not self-referred and can experience much of their lives as constraining. Thus, an explanation of the MI approach is even more important with these populations.

Tip for Opening Statement: Respond to Disbelief by Emphasizing Personal Choice

A possible response to the use of such an opening strategy is disbelief, particularly when the young person is in trouble with authorities. The youth may continue to lump you in with other authority figures with comments such as "I know you have to do your job and make me stop using" or "You have to make me follow the rules of probation." So, how you respond to statements of disbelief is critical and can shape the course of the encounter. Rather than taking these statements personally, or attempting to provide a rationale for treatment, you should provide an honest and forthright response that allows the young person to take responsibility for his or her decision to engage in the encounter (or not). For example, "I can't change what happened that made others think you need to be here, but I can help you explore what's going on and how you decide you want to handle it." You may also ask for clarification to further understand the young person's point of view. For example, "You expect people to make you do things. Tell me more about that."

Tip for Opening Statement: Be Careful with Intensity

Meynard (2008) suggests that while eye contact is typically considered a sign of active listening, eye contact that is too intense may make the young person uncomfortable. Simply displaying affect that is too intense or is inconsistent with the young person's affect, for example being too cheery, can also alienate a teen.

Another way of lessening discomfort is to reduce the use of words such as "you" or "your." Young persons can perceive these statements as blaming and derogatory, and subsequently experience anger toward you, as well as increase their avoidance of discussing relevant behavioral change issues. Thus, statements such as "You feel confused about why you are here," may be better received by depersonalizing the statement. Instead try, "Young people often feel confused about why they have to come here."

Tip for Opening Statement: Avoid the Term "Problem"

Avoiding the term "problem" is important, for this can be viewed as similar to a diagnosis or label; both carry a negative connotation and also decrease the young person's self-efficacy to effect change in his or her behavior. For example, young persons labeled as "alcoholic" may believe there is little they can do to alter their drinking, as it is a "problem" or "diagnosis" that cannot be changed. Instead, by simply naming the behavior, "you were referred to discuss drinking," you increase the conveyance of a nonjudgmental attitude, which will make the adolescent more likely to be open and honest.

Agenda Setting

After setting the tone of treatment with an opening statement, the spirit of collaboration can be expressed by agenda setting with the young person. Agenda setting can be as simple as offering the choice of what to discuss first, "Would you prefer to talk first about marijuana, alcohol, or what's going on in school?" A more thorough approach involves eliciting the young people's view of their concerns. Miller and Rollnick (2002) suggest asking the person about the concerns he or she would like to discuss. You can then also mention what you might like to talk about, and decide with the young person where to start.

Tip for Agenda Setting: Ask Permission

A primary strategy for conveying MI spirit in all encounters is to ask for permission before engaging in a task. Not only does asking permission show that you are respecting the young person's autonomy, it also serves to increase engagement as it requires the young person to verbally agree to engage in the task. This can be done as a preface for conversational tasks, "If it's OK with you, I would like to find out more about your substance use." It can also be done more formally for more intensive tasks such as written activities. For example, "Would you be willing for us to write down the behaviors we just agreed to focus on in our sessions?" Of course, the young person can always choose not to engage (i.e., say no after you ask for permission). While this negative response can be more than disappointing for you, it is ultimately more likely to increase alliance. When young persons see that you respect their decision not to engage in a task, they are more likely to believe the collaborative spirit you are trying to convey.

Tip for Agenda Setting: Use Visual Tools

Visual tools are an excellent way to engage young persons, particularly those who are less verbal. Examples include offering opportunities to draw or create art about the future, while discussing goals or creating a specific list of the characteristics important to what they wish their life would be like. An agenda-setting chart, originally described by Stott, Rollnick, and Pill (1995) and further explicated by Rollnick and colleagues (2008), is a visual collaborative tool for brief medical consultations. Channon, Huws-Thomas, Gregory, and Rollnick (2005) adapted the tool for teenagers with diabetes not only to set an agenda but also to develop a therapeutic alliance. In this adaptation, you explain that to best understand how the potentially problematic behavior fits in with the person's life, the young person can create a "sort of map" with different aspects of the behavior. The map is completed as the session progresses and can include other aspects of the young person's life that may be of importance. You can make the size of the circles reflect level of importance, and the circles can overlap. Other areas of interest that may not be on the treatment agenda can be written outside the circles. Figure 3.1 demonstrates a map from the case of Jenny struggling with obesity.

After the map is complete, you and the young person may then collaboratively decide on the agenda and potential goals of treatment. During this part of the process, it is important for you to consider focusing on short-term goals rather than only long-term outcomes. Short-term goals directly related to the behavior (e.g., not smoking cannabis during the week) or indirectly related to the behavior (e.g., increasing participation in after-school activities) may be initially more appealing than long-term goals (e.g., quitting) and may be more likely to lead to success. In addition, setting intermediary goals allows young persons to experience a sense of accomplishment and success in making changes, which can also increase their self-efficacy for continued engagement in change.

Typical-Day Exercise

Another helpful strategy, the typical-day exercise (Rollnick, Miller, & Butler, 2008), allows you to obtain information pertinent to setting a collaborative agenda for treatment and has been successfully utilized with adolescents (Channon et al., 2005). You ask the young person to walk through the activities, interactions, and associated feelings they experience in a typi-

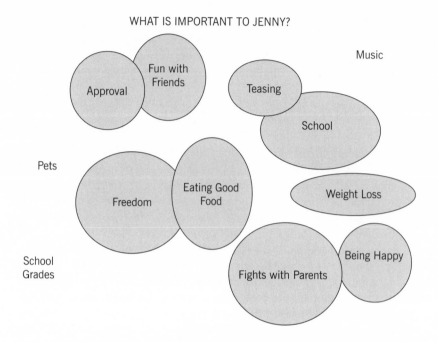

FIGURE 3.1. Agenda map for the case of Jenny.

cal day. For example, you might ask "think about yesterday and take me through it. Just tell me what happened, and, if you want, tell me how you felt about things." In using the typical-day exercise with young persons, it may be helpful to inquire about a weekday, as well as a weekend day, as behavioral routines can significantly differ. It is important to note that this technique differs from other behavioral assessment strategies, such as self-monitoring or time-sampling procedures, in which the identification of problematic behaviors and their associated consequences are targeted for intervention.

Tip for Typical Day: Explore What Is Important to the Young Person

When the young person seems hesitant to discuss the target behavior at all, an option is to explore other areas of the young person's life first. These details can appear unimportant at first glance; however they provide a critical opportunity to learn about the goals and values of the young person. Topics to consider inquiring about include peers ("Tell me what you usually like to do with your friends?"), family ("What do your parents typically do that drive you crazy?"), and school ("What do you like and not like about school?"). By allowing the young person to discuss these less risky and preferred topics, you continue to establish the bond of trust necessary for working with young persons. Furthermore, the young person may reveal other important intermediary goals that you would not have thought of, further supporting the notion that the young person is the expert of his or her life.

Providing Information: Elicit–Provide–Elicit or Ask–Tell–Ask

Often in the first session, you must convey certain basic information (e.g., confidentiality, length of treatment). Rollnick and colleagues (2008) suggest the technique of elicit–provide–elicit (EPE) when providing information or feedback. While this technique is discussed in later chapters in more detail, we briefly address EPE here as an opening strategy. First, your goal is to ask or *elicit* permission. The second step is to *provide* information. Last, you *elicit* the young person's point of view regarding the information provided such as "What do you make of that?", or "How does this sound to you?" As a point of reference, you should not provide more than two or three sentences of information without eliciting the person's thoughts or feelings about that information.

> PRACTITIONER: If it's OK with you, I would like to tell you about confidentiality. (Elicit)
>
> YOUNG PERSON: Sure.
>
> PRACTITIONER: Well, basically I won't share information you tell me unless it's about hurting yourself or someone else. And in those situations, we would talk about who I would need to tell and exactly what I would tell them. (Provide) What do you think of that? (Elicit)
>
> YOUNG PERSON: Well, I guess that makes sense. What do you mean by hurting myself?
>
> PRACTITIONER: If you told me that you were going to do something that put your life in danger, we would have to make a plan to tell someone else in your life to keep you safe. (Provide) Does that make sense? (Elicit)

SUMMARY

In our own training and practice, we have learned that MI is as often about what to refrain from saying or doing as it is about what to actually say or do in conversations with young people. Thus, we summarize each component of the pyramid by providing a table of suggested MI dos and don'ts consistent with the ACE themes of autonomy, collaboration, and evocation and the principles of expressing empathy, developing discrepancy, rolling with resistance, and supporting self-efficacy.

SUMMARY: MI DOS AND DON'TS—THE SPIRIT OF MI

What to do	What not to do
Support autonomy.	Take responsibility or take control.
Guide.	Prescribe.
Evoke intrinsic motivation and confidence.	Tell the young person why and how to change.
Create an atmosphere of warmth and acceptance.	Focus on behavior change or problem solving at the expense of expressing empathy.
Elicit discrepancy between the young person's goals/values and behavior.	Emphasize external demands or your reasons to change.
Actively listen and ride the wave of sustain talk.	Convince or interpret.
Promote behavior-specific optimism and hope.	Focus on global self-worth or inadvertently undermine self-efficacy by setting unrealistic goals.
Collaborate with the young person regarding the goals and tasks of treatment in the initial encounter.	Assume to know what is the "real" problem/diagnosis or to have the best ideas on how to fix the problem.

✳ ✳ ✳ ✳

Person-Centered Guiding Skills

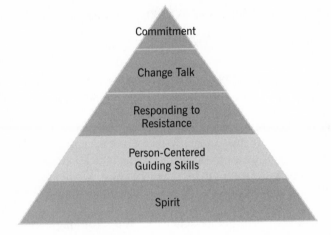

Listening is a magnetic and strange thing, a creative force. . . . When
we are listened to, it creates us, makes us unfold and expand. Ideas
actually begin to grow within us and come to life . . . and it is this
little creative fountain inside us that begins to spring and cast up new
thoughts and unexpected laughter and wisdom.
—BRENDA UELAND, *Strength to Your Sword Arm: Selected Writings*

Person-centered communication skills build upon the opening strategies
described in the previous chapter and provide a platform for conveying the
MI spirit for both the first and subsequent encounters. These skills specify
how to actively listen to the young person, help you to develop a greater
rapport and therapeutic alliance, and allow for the exploration of ambivalence guiding. Later chapters (see Chapters 6 and 7) discuss how you use

Person-centered communication skills build upon the opening strategies described in the previous chapter and provide a platform for conveying the MI spirit for both the first and subsequent encounters.

these skills to strategically guide the person toward change. The person-centered guiding skills are known by the mnemonic OARS—open-ended questions, affirmations, reflections, and summaries. We begin with reflections because they are the foundation of active listening.

REFLECTIONS: THE KEY TO BEING AN ACTIVE LISTENER

Reflective statements have many purposes. For the person-centered component of MI, reflections are used to communicate accurate empathy and to test your hypotheses about how the young person experiences the world (in Chapters 6 and 7 we discuss the goal-oriented component). Offering reflections involves stating to the person what you heard, possibly adding an emphasis or meaning. Miller and Rollnick (2002) assert that you cannot reflect too much, and this is usually true. One exception might be overly reflecting feelings of despair and helplessness, which may in turn reinforce negative thoughts and stifle further conversation. We next review the two broad categories of reflections for active listening: simple reflections and complex reflections. Under these categories, MI specifies several different types of reflections to promote active listening. You might consider these reflections as a menu of options from which to choose what feels most right to you in the moment. Sometimes you might want to do what feels comfortable, and sometimes you might want to try something new.

Simple Reflections

When you repeat or paraphrase the young person's words, you express understanding with a simple reflection. The reflection is "simple" because you do not add any specific meaning or emphasis on the content of what has been said. For example, when a young person says "I hate coming in here, how much longer do I have to come?" a paraphrase might sound like "You really don't want to come here." However, it is important to note that exact repetition of the young person's verbiage may engender a frustrated or sarcastic response, such as "that's what I just said." Thus, your goal should be to use exact repetition for only a part of the person's statement ("you hate it"), or you can also alternate your use of simple reflections with other types of more complex reflections described below.

Using reflections for the first time brings both challenges and rewards. As you begin to incorporate reflections into your repertoire, it can be common to wonder if they are sounding a bit contrived to the young person.

You may even feel a little clumsy as you begin to practice this new skill, similar to when you first learned to drive a car. When there is so much else to attend to, it can take a while to get comfortable and see the road ahead. When you offer a simple reflection to the young person, it is akin to handing over the steering wheel to the other person. While the idea of giving the keys of your car to a first-time driver can be disconcerting, we have learned that with time you can get better and better at allowing the young person to take control over the content of the MI.

If your simple reflection is met with silence, try to resist filling the silence immediately. Allow the young person the time to absorb the idea that you are offering him or her an invitation to continue to talk. Given that adolescents often perceive themselves as not being listened to, when you choose to offer the gift of a reflection, we find that your present will most always be received with open arms.

Complex Reflections

Miller and Rollnick (2002) specify several types of complex reflections. Do not worry about memorizing the names of each type of reflection. Instead, be aware that you can choose from a menu of options. Your choice of reflections will be guided by your comfort as well as the young person's communications with you.

A reflection of the person's *true meaning* expresses the implication of the person's statement. For example, if a young person is talking about the multiple appointments he has to attend because of his probation, you might respond with a statement such as "You are tired of people telling you what to do."

A *double-sided reflection* emphasizes ambivalence when you reflect both sides of the young person's mixed feelings about change. It serves to point out the discrepancy between the adolescent's values or goals for change, and how her behavior(s) may detract from helping her to attain these outcomes. When engaging in these reflections, Miller and Rollnick (2002) suggest using the conjunction "and" instead of "but" to further normalize having two simultaneously occurring feelings about the target behavior, as this ambivalence is commonly found in most persons seeking to make a change. For example, in the case of an adolescent who smokes cigarettes but is considering quitting, a double-sided reflection might sound like: "On the one hand you really like smoking, and on the other hand it is costing you a lot of money." With these types of reflections, it is also especially strategic to end with the positive side of change, as in the current example, since the person may be more likely to respond to the latter portion of your response.

After you have established rapport, you can begin to use reflection of *client feeling*—reflecting emotions the person either described or implied.

For example, in the case of an adolescent seeking to lose weight and expressing concerns about avoiding classes due to his weight, you might respond: "You're disappointed when you miss out on things like participating in sports or gym class because of your weight." While it can be a concern that young people may shy away from reflections of feeling, Resnicow (2008) notes that practitioners actually tend to underemphasize reflections of feeling because of their own personal fear of addressing emotions. We believe that for young people, the avoidance of experiencing uncomfortable emotions (such as fear or anger) can be at the core of ambivalence, and discussion of emotions may be necessary for change to occur. For example, Resnicow suggests, instead of offering the young person a more cognitive response, such as "you are concerned," you could use language that reflects more emotional content, such as "you are worried." As long as you are actually responding to what the young person has expressed or implied (and not straying too far from it), he or she still has the choice to either accept the reflection or clarify whether what you said was inaccurate.

When you reflect emotions, it is especially important to consider the timing of the reflection. For example, if rapport has not yet been established, a lower-intensity word (a little sad) may be better than a high-intensity word (really depressed). However, as adolescents are a heterogeneous group, you may also want to emphasize the most prevalent emotions discussed during the encounter, such as feeling anger about having to change. Take, for example, a young person who is bursting with emotions of anger, and how he might feel misunderstood if you say, "You were a little angry," if, in fact, they were "steaming mad."

Metaphors and similes are akin to painting a picture of the young person's experience. Specifically, metaphors and similes associate distinct but comparable emotions, ideas, and images. Similes, for example, typically incorporate the use of the word "like" or "as," such as "She is crazy like a fox." Metaphors and similes can be powerful in conveying a specific message to a young person, and can help him or her to view you as a person rather than just another helping professional who uses a lot of technical language. For example, when dealing with a young person who is court-mandated to treatment and tells you no one understands her, a statement such as "Everyone is on your back" can more quickly help you develop a deeper rapport than using jargon about the nuances of the treatment. You may also use a metaphor or simile to reflect on what is happening in real time in the session, "Sometimes it's like you want to rush through our sessions and not talk much. A speeding bullet that moves so fast you hardly notice it."

As in all reflections, it is important not to stray far from what the young person is conveying; otherwise, you will engender more resistance. Certainly, you may use metaphors or similes that the young person offers. However, we caution against using metaphors and similes that are not natural for you. For example, using what you think is a "cool metaphor" about topics such as skateboarding or rap music, when you really have no idea about the topic, will appear false to the young person. Instead, it is best to begin using these skills by discussing scenarios you and the young person both understand and that will facilitate (rather than hinder) a continued conversation about behavior change.

Tip for Reflections: Drop the Stems

It is common to begin reflections with stems such as "It sounds like . . ." or "So . . ." or "What you're saying is . . ." However, in most situations, it is generally preferable to drop the stem. The additional words are not necessary and take away more than they add to the content of the message. Moreover, we find that practitioners tend to overuse these stems in clinical encounters. Many adolescents will immediately shy away from statements such as "It sounds like you're feeling . . .," particularly when they have been seen by other practitioners who use this crutch. The stems make the discussion seem more like therapy than like a conversation. If you fall into the trap of overusing the same stem, it may foster nothing in the young person but utter annoyance with you.

Tip for Reflections: Avoid Turning Reflections into Questions

Inflection—how you use your tone of voice at the end of a statement (i.e., turning it up into a question or stating it in a neutral tone that smacks of a flat-sounding statement)—can make or break the impact of your reflection. Your goal should be to maintain a neutral inflection of tone in your use of reflections, as they can easily be turned into questions without careful monitoring. Turning reflections into closed-ended questions can suggest you are not listening and may be interpreted by the young person as judging their behavior. For example, if a person describes his drinking frequency, you might reflect, "You drank a case of beer" and lower the inflection to sound straightforward. If you say "You drank a case of beer?" the young person may feel judged because you sound surprised and even disappointed. Try this out loud and see how it sounds. As another example, in the case of a teenage girl who expresses sadness about her boyfriend's behavior, a neutral reflection, such as "You felt sad when your boyfriend did not show up," would be better received than if you said, "You felt sad?" By turning the reflection into a question you convey a sense of not really listening, and in the worst case, could give the impression that her feelings were invalid or unreasonable for the situation.

OPEN-ENDED QUESTIONS

While a significant amount of communication can occur from reflections alone, there will be times when the flow of conversation slows and a question can help elicit more of the person's views or concerns. In MI, you minimize closed-ended questions because they do not facilitate conversation. Rather, closed-ended questions usually elicit single-word responses. Furthermore, you will glean much more relevant information from open-ended questions. For example, recall the old game of 20 questions? One player thinks of a famous person, and the second player poses yes–no questions. It usually takes at least five questions to guess the answer. In contrast, one open-ended question such as, "Tell me what you have done in your life," can elicit enough information to guess the famous person.

Too many questions, however, can make the young person feel interrogated and can give the impression you are not listening to the answers. Moyers, Martin, Manuel, Hendrikson, and Miller (2005) suggest that a ratio of two reflections to every question is optimal to promote behavior change. One way to ensure this balance in your encounters is to use a reflective statement before and after every question.

> One way to ensure this balance in your encounters is to use a reflective statement before and after every question.

PRACTITIONER: You said that taking your medications makes you feel sick. (Reflection) What kinds of side effects do you feel? (Question)

YOUNG PERSON: Well, it makes me nauseous if I take it on an empty stomach and I don't like to eat in the morning.

PRACTITIONER: If you take your medicine with food, your stomach does not bother you, but the problem is figuring out how to do that in the morning. (Reflection)

The balance between the reflection–question–reflection allows for a more balanced conversation instead of coming across like an assessment or, at worst, an interrogation, which can easily lead to increased resistance. If you are required to do an intake or formal assessment early in the treatment process, balancing reflections and questions at this early point will help you convey the spirit of MI and enhance your collaborations with the young person.

Tip for Questions: Use Open-Ended Questions
to Facilitate Behavior Recognition

Certain open-ended questions can be particularly helpful for eliciting information from people who do not perceive themselves as having a problem. These questions center on inquiring about other people in the person's life and take the focus away from the young person. For example, questions you can include are: "What has happened that other people think you need to be here?" or "What is it that other people are concerned about?" or "What do other people hassle you about?"

Tip for Questions: Use Open-Ended Questions to Respond to Shocking Statements

Another use of open-ended questions is to respond to the young person telling you something controversial. Statements can include either a boasting about risk ("I've tried every drug on the planet"), a shocking statement ("I had sex with five girls yesterday"), or something they want you to keep from their parents but makes you uncomfortable ("I might be pregnant but don't tell my parents"). During these situations, responding with a question expressed with curiosity, not judgment, can be key ("How did you think I would react to that statement?"). Of course, you can always reflect, but by asking an open-ended question you elicit, rather than interpret, the meaning behind the statement. It also allows the young person to know you are paying attention, and solidifies his or her trust in you.

Tip for Questions: Consider Multiple-Choice Questions

There are also times when a young person may be stymied in the face of a very open-ended question such as "What do you make of all this?" Moreover, we have found that more resistant adolescents do not like to answer these types of questions. An alternative to open-ended questions in these situations is to provide a multiple-choice question, such as "Do you feel upset by this, fine with it, or maybe something else?" In this way, you provide structure for the conversation while still offering choice.

AFFIRMATIONS

According to the *Merriam-Webster Online Dictionary*, to *affirm* means not only to state positively, but also to validate and confirm something the young person has already said. Sue (2008) wrote about the concept of affirmations as gift giving—a present you offer to show respect for the young person's strengths, as well as to increase positive feelings about the interaction. The key to affirmations is your use of honesty and specificity. We suggest that you not use generic affirmations that may ring false, such as in the classic *Saturday Night Live* parody on self-help when Stuart Smalley says to himself, "I am good enough, I'm smart enough, and dog-gone it, people like me." A more challenging young person may disengage from those generic, cheerleader-type statements. However, affirmations that target a specific strength or effort, and that (like reflections) are close to what the person has already said, are generally accepted. For example, instead of "You're smart," try "It's smart that you are thinking of your options."

It is also possible that an affirmation may engender sustain talk when a more challenging young person feels you are overly enthusiastic about change. For example, when you say "I am really happy you decided to cut back on your drinking," the young person may rebelliously stop the change process. To avoid this pitfall, affirmations alternatively can be framed without the use of "I" statements, such as "It's great that you decided to cut back on your drinking."

Tip for Affirmations: Consider the Timing

Careful consideration of the timing of your affirmation can guide the type of affirmation you choose. Affirmations about a specific behavior may be more acceptable when the person is more ready to change ("It's great that you want to cut back on your drinking"), whereas affirming strengths and values may be more beneficial when the person is less ready to change ("You are willing to consider difficult decisions in order to make the best choice for yourself"). Or you may only choose to use affirmations sparingly when a young person adamantly displays an opposition to treatment, and instead roll with resistance (see Chapter 5). Obviously, there is no single correct way of affirming a person. Rather, the key to affirmations, as in all person-centered skills, is to stay close to the person's communication and to be accurately focused on the person's response to your statements.

SUMMARIES

We have covered open-ended questions, affirmations, and the foundation of active listening—reflections. The last skill in OARS is summarizing. Miller and Rollnick (2002) describe this process as picking flowers and presenting them back to the person in a bouquet. Your goal is to select statements from the conversation and "connect the dots," by incorporating and preferably ending with motivating statements. For example, "You have told me a lot about why you like using marijuana. It helps you relax, and it is easier for you to have fun with your friends. You also said you have gotten into a lot of trouble because dope is illegal and it has started to cost you a lot of money. You are not sure you want to stop smoking marijuana right now, but you're wondering about what it's costing you."

Summaries such as this demonstrate to the young person that you are listening intently. Summaries also help a young person with limited abstract thinking abilities to pull together different pieces of the puzzle ("Let's stop for a minute and go over what we've discussed so far . . ."), help you to remember all these pieces ("So to make sure that I'm understanding everything correctly . . ."), and let you transition to different tasks of treatment or other components of the agenda ("We've covered a lot of topics, getting back to your goals for treatment . . .").

SUMMARY

Person-centered counseling skills begin to put MI principles into practice. We have elaborated on four person-centered counseling skills (OARS) to ensure empathy and active listening. What, if any, of these skills will you try out today either in practice or in your personal relationships?

SUMMARY: MI DOS AND DON'TS— PERSON-CENTERED GUIDING SKILLS

What to do	What not to do
Collaborate with the young person regarding the goals and tasks of treatment.	Assume to have the best ideas, how to fix the problem, or what is the *real* problem (or diagnosis).
Vary types of reflections without use of inflections.	Reflect only one side of the ambivalence, turn reflections into questions, overuse the same stem (e.g., "sounds like").
Balance open-ended and multiple-choice questions with reflections.	Be pressured into the question–answer–question–answer trap.
Affirm specific strengths and abilities to support self-efficacy.	Use generic affirmations (e.g., "Good job!") or be overenthusiastic of behavior change too quickly.
Summarize periodically to present a collection of reflections, to link themes, or to transition to other foci.	Stray too far from the person's statements.

CHAPTER 5

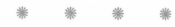

Responding to Resistance

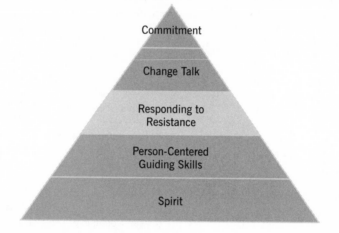

Then again, maybe I won't.
—Judy Blume

In the previous chapter, we focused on the person-centered component of
MI in terms of developing rapport and exploring the young person's point
of view. Before moving on to goal-directed techniques, we address the issue
of how to use reflections and other strategies to respond to young people
who are hesitant to collaborate with you, or who are not ready to work on
behavior change (both are common in young people who are not attending
treatment by their own volition). As noted in Chapter 3 (on MI spirit), an
MI approach considers resistance an *interpersonal* process, and, for adolescents and young adults, resistance is a *normal* developmental process
that results in three types of communication. First, you may hear "resistance talk," which can loosely be defined as negative comments about treat-

ment ("I don't need to come here") or about the relationship with you ("You will never understand what it's like for me"). Second, you will likely hear "sustain talk," which reflects statements about sustaining a behavior and not engaging in change. This language includes statements about

> An MI approach considers resistance an *interpersonal* process, and, for adolescents and young adults, resistance is a *normal* developmental process.

intentions not to change, ("You can tell me all you want, I'm not going to stop drinking with my friends"), the advantages of the status quo, ("If I stop drinking, my friends will all think I'm a loser"), disadvantages of change, ("All my friends drink. Who am I supposed to hang out with if I stop drinking?"), and pessimism about change, (i.e., "It doesn't matter, I tried to stop before, and none of the psychobabble the counselor told me helped)" Third, resistance or hesitancy about behavior change may also be represented by a lack of conversation (e.g., silence, telegraphic speech, or asking "huh?").

As outcome research on MI has evolved, we have learned that increases in motivational statements (later referred to as "change talk") are associated with behavior change in adults. However, with young people, an interesting phenomenon occurs. Reductions in sustain talk appear to be even more related to behavior change than are increases in motivational statements (Baer et al., 2008). Thus, we now turn our attention to ways to respond to reduce all three types of communication (resistance talk, sustain talk, and lack of conversation) in the spirit of MI.

RECOGNIZE RESISTANCE IN THE RELATIONSHIP

Your first step in responding to resistance is to recognize the interpersonal tension. Keeping with the fire analogy of "stop, drop, and roll" (see Chapter 3 on MI spirit), you must learn to recognize the first signs of smoke. Are you hearing negative comments about treatment or hesitation about engaging with you? Is the young person arguing with you about not needing to change? Are you feeling frustrated with the young person's silence? We ask you to think about how these comments fit on the continuum of clean air to the smoke in a full-fledged fire, and we then offer some tips for how you might go about keeping the embers at bay.

STEP BACK

Once you are aware of the burning situation, the second step is to monitor your own behavior and step back or drop down. It is difficult for a young person to fight against a practitioner who maintains a neutral stance and offers an appreciation of the dilemma of change. Wrestling requires two people, and if you stop, the young person cannot continue to wrestle. Recall that psychological reactance occurs in response to a perceived threat, and none of us responds well to a threat. You diminish reactance by becoming less threatening in your communication.

Tip for Stop, Drop, and Roll: Avoid Persuasion

Falling into a persuading or directing mode can be tempting, especially when the consequences of not changing are dire. However, what we have learned is that the more you try to persuade, the more the young person resists. Sometimes this persuasion can take the form of rescuing when you offer support and encouragement (i.e., "I know you can do it!") or when you direct ideas for change ("How about you try . . .") before the person is ready to listen to your ideas. Usually, you will experience what we call the "Yeah buts . . ." The young person will offer reasons why these ideas will not work, "Yeah, but I've tried that before." In fact, resistance is often the result of overestimating the young person's readiness to change. In addition to increasing sustain talk, another danger of persuasion is that the young person will respond with agreement without meaning ("OK, fine, I'll try it"), and no action or change actually occurs after the encounter is completed. As Rollnick and colleagues (2008, p. 148) state, "a good guide never gets too far in front."

PERSON-CENTERED GUIDING SKILLS TO RESPOND TO RESISTANCE

Simple Reflection

The simplest way to respond to resistance talk is with a simple reflection. Because most young people expect adults to respond to their statements with direction or persuasion, a reflection often stops them in their tracks.

> The simplest way to respond to resistance talk is with a simple reflection. Because most young people expect adults to respond to their statements with direction or persuasion, a reflection often stops them in their tracks.

YOUNG PERSON: I have no idea why I am here. (Resistance Talk) I don't have a drinking problem. (Sustain Talk)

PRACTITIONER: Your drinking is not a concern for you right now. (Reflection)

If delivered with genuineness and curiosity, a simple reflection often invites the person to elaborate, giving both parties time to consider a more constructive topic of conversation.

Omission Reflection

Omission reflections (Resnicow & McMaster, in press) can be helpful when you are responding to resistance that is represented nonverbally by a lack of communication. For example, to the young person who speaks little or responds with few words ("I'm fine"), you can respond by pointing out the message the nonverbal behavior suggests ("You're not sure if you want to talk to me about this"). You may also reflect on an omission of behavior change conversation to encourage more active discussion ("I notice you have not mentioned the reason your parents brought you here—your drug use. I am curious why you have not mentioned it?"). However, be prepared to step back if the response is further resistance (e.g, "It's not a problem for me").

Amplified Reflection

In an amplified reflection, you emphasize and intensify the sustain talk in the reflection, "There is no reason at all for you to take your HIV medications." If your tone is straightforward and honest, then these reflections will often elicit, "Yeah, but" statements followed by reasons to change. In this way, you evoke motivation from the young person instead of providing the rationale for them. In the example above, the young person may respond, "Yeah but the doctor says that my HIV virus is growing." Now, you may reflect the young person's potential reason for change, "Stopping the virus from growing may be a reason to take medications."

Amplified reflections can be tricky, and we emphasize that you must convey an attitude of empathy and not sarcasm. Too extreme of an overstatement or a reflection in the form of a question may elicit further resistance, particularly in young people who are well known to use sarcasm in their own daily communication repertoires. For example, "There is no reason at all to slow down your drinking?" may be experienced as judgmental and set you back from furthering the discussion.

Tip for Amplified Reflections: Try a Minimizing Reflection

Like amplified reflections that somewhat overstate sustain talk, minimizing reflections understate the reasons for change or the problems the person has had because of not changing. Minimizing reflections are also meant to increase the likelihood of the young person responding with arguments for change.

YOUNG PERSON: I don't know why they made me come here. (Resistance Talk) I drink for fun, but have never had a car accident. (Sustain Talk)

PRACTITIONER: You've only had a few really minor difficulties as a result of your drinking. (Minimizing Reflection)

YOUNG PERSON: Yeah, but these probation appointments are a real hassle. (Change Talk; see Chapter 5)

Tip for Amplified Reflections: Come Alongside
When the Young Person Agrees

If a young person responds to amplified and minimizing reflections with agreement instead of arguing for the other side of ambivalence (e.g., You're right, I have not had any problems from drinking"), there is still nothing lost. What the agreement offers you is a greater understanding of the depth of the young person's attachment to the status quo behavior. At this point, it may be wise to "come alongside" and reflect that now may not be the time to change ("Slowing down on your drinking isn't really anything you want or need to do right now"). The young person may then argue for the opposite, such as why it might be time to change, or you may collaboratively decide to focus on other behaviors (see the section, "Agenda Setting" in Chapter 3).

Tip for Amplified Reflections: Consider Using a Stem When Necessary

Amplifying, minimizing, and coming alongside are not paradoxical interventions, for they involve prescribing a behavior that is in opposition to change. However, younger adolescents and those who tend to be more concrete in their thinking may take your reflections of reasons not to change literally and mistake your statements as agreeing they should not change. Similarly, a more oppositional adolescent may tell others you condoned a behavior because you used these reflective statements. In these cases, it might be necessary to add a personalized stem, such as "You're saying . . ." or "I'm hearing . . ." to the reflection to prevent these misperceptions (e.g., "I'm hearing that you feel now may not be the right time to change")

STRATEGIC RESPONSES

We now describe four other strategies to respond to interpersonal resistance talk and sustain talk, which do not rely on OARS per se but still convey the spirit of MI.

Emphasizing Personal Control

The struggle for autonomy is most salient in adolescence, and the strategy of emphasizing person control can be most effective with this age group. With this strategy, your goal is to respond to resistance talk or sustain talk by emphasizing that it is really the person's right to choose whether or not to change. The strategy is a continuation of the opening statement (see Chapter 2) when the practitioner emphasized that pressuring people to change is counterproductive and that the practitioner's role is one of guiding. Below is an example from our case of Jenny struggling with weight loss.

> JENNY: I don't think I have a problem with my eating. I eat a lot of fruit, and all my friends eat as much as I do. (Sustain Talk)
>
> PRACTITIONER: It is really your choice about whether or not you are going to change your eating. Your parents can force some things, like what food they bring into the house, but they can't watch you all the time. It has to be your decision. (Emphasizing Personal Control)

Tip for Emphasizing Personal Control: Emphasize Choice in Highly Constrained or Dire Situations

Often young people's choices are quite constrained, as they are not yet legally allowed to make decisions for themselves. Furthermore, some behaviors may have dire consequences if they are illegal, or if the youth is in a particularly constraining environment, such as a detention facility or hospital. However, you can still offer choice opportunities, even if the consequences may be severe. For example, "I realize you will have to deal with whatever consequences are in place, but it is your choice whether or not to follow your probation plan." Alternatively, you can find places within the constraining environment where the young person can choose. For example, in the case of a young person with anorexia who is on a mandatory feeding program, the young person may be able to choose which feeding supplements to begin.

Pros and Cons

The pros and cons strategy is in some ways an elaboration of the double-sided reflection (see Chapter 4), but it can be used even if the young person is not expressing both sides of the ambivalence. The first step is to respond to sustain talk by asking for elaboration. For example, if the young person says, "I have no reason to quit marijuana," you may respond, "Tell me more about the things you like about using marijuana." By first eliciting the reasons for the status quo behavior, you can establish rapport, roll with resistance, and further understand the barriers to behavior change. After reflecting or summarizing the young person's view, we find that you can now safely ask for the pros of the behavior (e.g., taking medications or exercise), without eliciting resistance. However, if you ask for the pros of behavior change first, increased resistance may be more likely to occur.

Tip for Pros and Cons: Focus on Adopting a Positive Behavior
versus Avoiding a Negative Behavior

Because young people do not respond well to discussing the cons of a behavior that others want them to avoid, we suggest focusing on the pros and cons of adopting a new behavior (Moore & Parsons, 2000; Nickoletti & Taussig, 2006). Thus, for young people, the strategy is more aptly called "cons and pros." This adaptation works easily when the focus is on a health behavior, such as taking medication for a chronic illness or beginning an exercise regime. In using this strategy, you would first ask about the cons, or the bad things about the new positive behavior (i.e., "Tell me the not so good things about exercising"). After reflecting or summarizing the young person's view, you can then ask for the pros of the behavior (i.e., "What are the good things that happen when you exercise?"). When the goal is the avoidance of a behavior such as substance use, you can focus on the new behavior of "staying clean" rather than on the bad aspects of substance use. You begin by asking about the cons of staying clean, followed by the pros of quitting or cutting back. As always, we ask for permission to respect autonomy:

> PRACTITIONER: If it's OK with you, I would like to understand more about your view of the situation. I am wondering, what are the bad things about quitting smoking? (Eliciting the Cons of Change)
>
> YOUNG PERSON: Well, smoking helps me when I am stressed out. It's something I like to do at parties. (Sustain Talk)
>
> PRACTITIONER: It helps you to relax, and it is something you like to do with your friends. What else do you like about smoking? (Reflection, Question)
>
> YOUNG PERSON: That's about it. (Diminishing Sustain Talk)
>
> PRACTITIONER: OK. On the other side, what might be some reasons for quitting or cutting back on your smoking? (Eliciting the Pros of Change)
>
> YOUNG PERSON: Hmm. Well, I guess it might save me some money. (Change Talk; see Chapter 6)

Tip for Pros and Cons: When the Young Person Cannot Express the Pros of Behavior Change

If the young person is not able to come up with the pros of behavior change on his or her own, you can continue to roll with this ambivalence by using reflections (i.e., "So right now you are not sure there are any reasons to change") or by trying one of the other three strategies listed here. For example, another option if resistance is not too strong is to offer possible pros using elicit–provide–elicit (only after a thorough, empathic discussion of Cons).

> PRACTITIONER: If you would like to hear them, I have some pros other kids have mentioned about using condoms. (Elicit)
>
> YOUNG PERSON: Sure, I guess so.
>
> PRACTITIONER: Some kids have found they can protect themselves from catching other sexually transmitted infections, or that they can make sure they don't get someone pregnant. Others have mentioned they use fun condoms such as ones with flavors or special lubricants. (Provide) What do you think about these pros? (Elicit)
>
> YOUNG PERSON: I am not sure about the fun condoms, but I don't want to catch herpes—that would suck! (Change Talk; see Chapter 6)

Agreement with a Twist

In the agreement with a twist strategy, you seek to respond to sustain talk by first reflecting the young person's perspective, followed by reframing the statement with a new meaning that supports change. In this way, you validate their perspective, while still offering something new, such as a hint toward behavior change or optimism about change. Common examples include offering a possible direction for change, reframing by offering hope, and using an educational reframe.

As an example of giving a *possible direction for change*:

> YOUNG PERSON: I really don't know why my parents keep staying on my back. I wish they would leave me alone! (Sustain Talk)
>
> PRACTITIONER: Your parents are really driving you crazy. (Reflection) I wonder if there is some way we can make all this attention they give you more supportive. (Reframe)

As an example of reframing by *offering hope*:

YOUNG PERSON: I have tried to quit cigarettes so many times. Nothing works. There is no way I can do it. (Sustain Talk)

PRACTITIONER: I am hearing your frustration, but I am also seeing your persistence. You seem to be a person who keeps trying even when it's hard. (Reframe)

As an example of an *educational* reframe:

YOUNG PERSON: I can really hold my liquor. I can drink a six pack and still feel totally normal. (Sustain Talk)

PRACTITIONER: You feel like alcohol has little effect on you. (Reflection) I am not sure if you have heard this, but after people have been drinking for a while, the body gets used to the alcohol and it needs more and more to get drunk. (Reframe)

Shifting Focus

If other strategies do not help to reduce resistance or ongoing sustain talk, you may always shift the conversation focus away from sustaining the status quo behavior. We do not mean you should shift away or ignore relevant therapeutic content (e.g., discussing a sports team). Rather, you should steer the conversation around the stumbling blocks to other areas of therapeutic discussion. Options for shifting may include a discussion of other areas of the person's life that may be related to behavior change or an intermediary goal. You may also include a simple reassuring statement to let the young person know you do not have to focus on something he or she is not ready to discuss.

YOUNG PERSON: I do not want to take medication. (Sustain Talk) I know that's what you are going to tell me to do, and I am not going to do it. (Resistance Talk)

PRACTITIONER: I don't think it makes sense to tell you to do something when I don't know the whole story. Why don't you tell me more about what is going on with your health right now. (Shifting Focus)

SUMMARY

In this chapter, we defined interpersonal resistance and sustain talk. We also elaborated on the principle of "stop, drop, and roll" by describing reflective and strategic responses to resistance and sustain talk. Which of these strategies will you consider trying when you feel like you are wrestling with a young person or smelling smoke? What traps do you think you will find yourself in, and how do you think you might avoid them?

SUMMARY: MI DOS AND DON'TS— RESPONDING TO RESISTANCE

What to do	What not to do
Stop, drop, and roll.	Convince, persist, or advise.
Use different types of reflections to respond to resistance or sustain talk.	Argue against sustain talk, attempt to correct it, or fall into persuasion.
Respond strategically by emphasizing person control, agreeing with a twist, eliciting pros and cons, or shifting focus.	Ignore or avoid the young person's perspective (expressed by resistance talk or sustain talk) or continue to reflect when the conversation remains stuck.

CHAPTER 6

❋   ❋   ❋   ❋

Change Talk

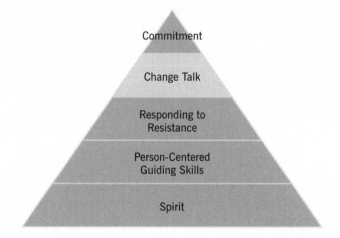

You have brains in your head
You have feet in your shoes
You can steer yourself any direction you choose.
Oh the places you'll go!

—Dr. Seuss

By rolling with resistance and using strategies to diminish sustain talk, you pave the way for the young person to take the first steps toward change. In this chapter, we move to the goal-oriented methods for encouraging young persons to continue in their journey of change (Channon et al., 2005). In the previous chapter, we discussed how to respond to sustain talk (intentions not to change, advantages of the status quo, disadvantages of change, and pessimism about change). We now discuss how to reinforce the young person's motivational statements called change talk (intentions to change, disadvantages of the status quo, advantages of change, and optimism about change).

THE FIRST FEW MILES IN THE JOURNEY OF CHANGE

In the first few miles of the journey of change, you will hear change talk without strong commitment. These are expressions of the young person's desires, abilities, reasons, and needs to alter the unhealthy behavior. Statements of desire begin with words such as "I want," "I wish," "I am motivated," and "I would like to." Statements about ability to change convey confidence but do not have to include a declaration of readiness, such as "I think I could do that, but I am not sure I am ready to." Typical stems include "I could," "I am able to," and "It's possible." Desire and ability statements may also take the form of things the young person has tried to do: "I tried to talk to my boyfriend about condoms." Regardless of the success of the attempt, the act of trying indicates motivation and is considered change talk.

Statements of need add a sense of urgency to the situation and consist of words such as "I need," "I must," "I have to," "I have got to," and "I cannot keep doing this." Statements about reasons for change can include desire and need, but add specificity to the content. Thus, reason statements can indicate that the young person may be less ambivalent and further along in the journey of change. For example, a statement such as "I have to do this" conveys a need to change. In contrast, a reason statement would convey a need paired with a specific rationale for the change. For example, "I need to do this for *my health*."

Tip: Don't Worry If Reasons for Change Are Unrealistic

Remember, the young person's reasons for change may not be consistent with yours or that of other adults. The reasons may also not be realistic (e.g., "I need to quit smoking so I can play professional basketball"), and you may even be tempted to laugh at the rationales some young people offer (e.g., "I need to cut back on drinking so I can save my money for this new video game"). It is important to maintain a nonjudgmental stance and recognize this really does not matter since the end result is increased motivation for change.

> Remember, the young person's reasons for change may not be consistent with yours or that of other adults.

REINFORCING CHANGE TALK TO CONTINUE THE JOURNEY

When you have learned to recognize change talk, how do you respond to it? Person-centered guiding skills are used to selectively respond and reinforce change talk. We first provide an example of OARS responses to change talk woven within a typical conversation with a young person. We then explain each strategy in further detail. In the case of Jenny struggling with following a weight-loss plan:

> JENNY: My mother moans at me all the time, and it's not as easy as she thinks. If she got off my back I might do a lot better (Ability to Change), but the arguments we have are just too much, they just make me want to eat more.
>
> PRACTITIONER: You might do a lot better with following your eating plan if you and your mother would stop fighting. (Reflection of Ability)
>
> JENNY: Yeah, all day long she hassles me about what I ate. It makes me want to just quit this whole thing, but I really want to lose some weight before summer. (Desire for Change)
>
> PRACTITIONER: Tell me more about why you want to lose weight before summer. (Question to Elaborate Change Talk)
>
> JENNY: All the kids hang out outside in shorts and t-shirts. When it is hot, I won't go because I don't want to wear clothes to show my fat. (Reasons for Change)
>
> PRACTITIONER: It's great that you want to lose weight so that you can go outside and be with the other kids. (Affirmation of Reasons for Change) What ideas do you have about what we could ask your parents to do to support you instead of fighting with you so that you reach your goal? (Open-Ended Question)
>
> JENNY: Well, she just needs to leave me alone because I really need to make this plan work. (Need for Change) Maybe she could just check in with me at the end of the day, but I am not sure she would do it.
>
> PRACTITIONER: You have some great ideas here. (Affirmation) When you fight with your mom, you want to eat more. This upsets you because you really want to lose weight so that you are more comfortable hanging out with your friends this summer. If we could talk to your mother about only checking in with you about eating only at the end of the day, it might help you achieve your goal. (Summary)

Reflections

When in doubt, reflect the change talk! For example, if a young person remains hesitant to try out a new behavior, but offers a statement about ability to change ("I know what to do to cut back on smoking, but I am not sure I am ready"), you reinforce the change talk embedded in ambivalence by reflecting it, "You really believe you can do this."

Tip: Don't Hesitate to Use the Word "You" When Reflecting Change Talk

When describing opening strategies in Chapter 3, we emphasized caution in the overuse of statements beginning with "you" as they may increase the young person's reactance early in the change process. However, when reflecting change talk, the incorporation of "you" statements, as in the examples above, clearly emphasizes personal choice in the change process. By maintaining this continued collaboration throughout the encounter (and not only during the initial rapport building phase), you can enhance the young person's sense of self-efficacy and continue to set the stage for behavior change.

Tip: Use Action Reflections to Address Ambivalence in Change Talk

In the early stages of the journey of change, ambivalence is not resolved. Jenny, the teen struggling with obesity, might say, "I would be able to lose weight if my mom stopped nagging me." Another example could be, "I tried to talk to her about helping me lose weight, but she just does not get it." The ambivalent young person will often follow change talk with an undermining statement, but this should not lead you away from reinforcing the change talk in the statement. You can address the barriers after you reinforce the change talk. In an action reflection (Resnicow & McMaster, in press), you reflect what the person says in a way that suggests a potential future action toward behavior change. For example, "you think you can follow your meal plan if we can find a way to have your mother stick to checking in only once a day." An affirming response with an action reflection is, "It's great that you have tried to talk to your mother to reduce the fights. If we can come up with a way for her to really understand you, it might work." The practitioner reflects the change talk and the ambivalence, and ends the statement with a possible action to be discussed later during the goal setting process.

Open-Ended Question to Elaborate Change Talk

When a young person makes a change talk statement, you can ask for elaboration with questions, such as "Tell me more about that." Another more specific request for elaboration used with a young person with alcohol issues might sound like: "You say now might be a time to consider cutting back on alcohol. How would you go about it if you were ready?" Note that the content of these questions closely parallels the subject matter of the young person's statements, without moving ahead too quickly to change topics or begin behavioral change planning.

Tip: Avoid Asking for Elaboration about Steps and Plans at Earlier Stages of Change Talk

In this early phase of the journey, where change talk does not include a commitment (see Chapter 7), be cautious in using direct questions about next steps and plans. For instance, in the previous example, the practitioner adds the caveat "if you were ready," in order to reduce the young person's perception of being pushed into discussing actions or taking steps for which he or she is not truly ready. In addition, prefacing the question with a reflection is another way you can mirror the young person's statements, to help guide alongside instead of stepping ahead. "You are considering cutting back on alcohol but you are not sure now is the right time. How might you go about doing it when you are ready?"

Affirmations

Affirmations often flow naturally from change talk statements and as always should be closely tied to the content of the change talk. Affirmations may be incorporated even when you are not directly affirming behavior change. In the earlier case of Jenny, the practitioner affirms her reasons for change even though she is not describing actual behavior change in terms of weight loss. Here is another example of the practitioner using caution when affirming a young person who is early in the change process. The young person says, "I keep having these horrible hangovers when I drink. That might be a reason to slow down." Instead of prematurely affirming behavior change, "It is wonderful that you are considering cutting back on your drinking," the practitioner affirms the patient's strengths, "You seem to be aware of your body's reaction to drugs. You really know yourself."

Summaries

Summaries may be used for the purpose of stringing together several change talk statements, addressing existing ambivalence, and guiding toward change by ending the summary in that direction. In the case of Jenny, the practitioner summarizes her struggle, highlighting change talk without ignoring ambivalence and ending with a direction for change.

Summaries may be especially relevant for young people, for they may be more prone to impulsively stating contradictory change and sustain talk statements in the same conversation, particularly in the face of ongoing ambivalence. For example, the young person who has been drinking and smoking cannabis daily may offer change talk at the beginning of the encounter, "I'm going to quit!" but minutes later respond with sustain talk, "What was I thinking, there is no way I can do this." While change talk may seem fleeting and consistency at times a rarity, a summary can help connect the dots in a positive way. You can go beyond merely stringing together change talk statements, and begin to tip the balance of pros and cons of behavior change. For example, "You mentioned a few concerns about taking antidepressants. Though you are not sure you want to put any more chemicals inside your body, you mentioned your mood is better when you take your medication, and you seem to have more energy. While you are not sure you really want to take these medications for the rest of your life, you are wondering if there might be some short-term benefit."

QUESTIONS TO ELICIT CHANGE TALK

You will often hear spontaneous change talk when actively listening to the young person's point of view. However, at times you may not hear change talk at all. We find this is particularly common among young people who are very ambivalent. You may be able to reduce resistance talk and sustain talk with the strategies in Chapter 4, but at the same time may find that the conversation does not automatically tilt to change talk. We now present adaptations of open-ended questions to elicit change talk and to guide the young person to maximize his or her potential. As always, you will want to reinforce any resulting change talk with OARS, and listen carefully for any reemergence of resistance signaling that you have moved too quickly.

Direct Questions

Perhaps the most direct way to elicit change talk is to ask for it (see Table 6.1 for sample questions). For example, "If you decided to make a change, how would you do it?" or "What difficulties have you experienced with your diabetes?" Emphasizing your interest in the young person's perceptions and not rehashing other's opinions about "what" and "how" they should change can facilitate this process, (i.e., "What do you think needs to change in your life?", or "I am interested in what *you* think. What concerns you about your drug use?").

> PRACTITIONER: Everyone is telling you what needs to change. What do *you* want? What part of your life feels less than perfect for you right now?
>
> YOUNG PERSON: Well, I suppose my life would be better if my parents would get off my back. (Change Talk)

TABLE 6.1. Examples of Change Talk

Preparatory change talk: DARN	Sounds like . . .
Desire: want, wish, like	• "I want to stop smoking; you don't know how hard it is." • "I wish I could lose some weight to be thin like everyone else." • "I would like to follow my parents' rules so they wouldn't nag so much."
Ability: can, could, able	• "I can take my medicine on my own without my parents reminding me all of the time." • "I could cut back on the weed if I wanted to." • "I might be able to cut back on sweets on weekends."
Reason: specific reason for change	• "I really don't want to end up on dialysis." • "If I get another dirty UA, they'll kick me out of this place."
Need: have to, must, important (without stating specific reason)	• "I need to lose some serious weight." • "I've got to get my blood sugar totally down from where it is."

PRACTITIONER: So you might consider making a change if it would reduce the hassle you experience with your parents. What would it take to make that happen? (Reflection, Elaboration)

Tip for Direct Questions: Tailor Questions with What You Already Know

By tailoring questions to elicit change talk based on what you already have learned about the young person, you further convey empathy and tie together the person-centered and goal-oriented components of MI. For example, in the case of Jenny, you might say, "You mentioned earlier that you tend to eat more when your mother fights with you. What do you think needs to change here?"

Tip for Direct Questions: Ask about Other People's Concerns When the Young Person Refuses to Acknowledge Any

Inquiring about how others perceive the problem behavior can elicit change talk. You can then follow up with reflections, and explore any sense of uneasiness they may be experiencing, drawing parallels between how others feel and their own views about change.

PRACTITIONER: What is it about your behavior that other people might see as a reason for concern?"

YOUNG PERSON: Well I don't think they have a reason, but my parents are worried my weight will mess up my health.

PRACTITIONER: So your parents are worried about you.

YOUNG PERSON: Yeah, they keep saying I might get diabetes like my father.

Now the practitioner can tie others' concerns to the young person's point of view.

PRACTITIONER: So they care about you and are worried about diabetes since there is a family history. What do you think?

YOUNG PERSON: Well, I am fine right now but I guess sometimes I wonder if I might end up like him down the road. (Change Talk)

PRACTITIONER: There is a part of you that wonders if you will end up with diabetes because of your weight, though perhaps not right away. (Reflection)

Alternatively, if others' concerns are not sufficient to elicit a discussion about the young person's potential reasons to change, some young people respond to questions that consider the effects of the target behavior on significant others.

YOUNG PERSON: I am fine right now, and I wish they [parents, friends] would not worry so much.

PRACTITIONER: So you are not sure this is an issue, but you don't like them [parents, friends] worrying. What could you do to reduce their worry?

YOUNG PERSON: Well, I guess I could consider eating healthier, but I am not going on a diet. (Change Talk)

PRACTITIONER: So if you could figure out a way to eat healthier without using a structured diet, it might work. (Action Reflection)

Imagining Questions

By discussing imagined situations, you can explore the young person's goals and guide them to the path of change talk. Imagining extremes involves asking future-oriented questions pertaining to how life would be if the problematic behavior continues and/or is discontinued. For example,

"What's the worst thing that might happen if you continue (insert problem behavior)?" and "What's the best thing that might happen if you decided to stop (insert problem behavior)?" Answers to these scenarios often resound of change talk. If the response is "nothing," consider this to be evidence of resistance in the relationship and roll with it (see Chapter 5).

A similar imagining approach involves asking the young person to imagine his or her life before the problem behavior existed. For example, "Looking back, tell me what your life was like before you started drinking." When inquiring about the past, you should allow for ample time to answer, and particularly for those young persons with a history of struggling to change the problematic behavior. Topics brought forth can provide new insights about what is actually important to the young person (and not just what you assumed). These topics can range from discussions about life being simpler as a child or experiencing less conflict with parents to noticing differences in appearance, health, and the like.

You can also ask the young person to look ahead by envisioning hopes for the future and considering how their current behaviors can help or hinder goal attainment. For example, "If you could be like an MP3 player and fast forward to when you are an adult, what would you see yourself doing, and how does your (problem behavior) fit with that goal, assuming nothing changes?" If the young person is not able to see that far ahead, try shorter windows of time, "What would your life look like one year from now?"

We have found the looking forward strategy to be especially powerful because it instills hopefulness about how life may one day be different. However, we have also found this strategy to backfire, increasing the young person's resistance if you are not prepared to roll with *any and all* responses he or she may offer. For all of us working with young persons, it is easy to slip into the trap of giving unsolicited advice (i.e., warning about the hazards of their ideas, such as responding with statements as "You'll end up in the hospital if you don't . . . "). However, these well-intentioned warnings often do little but evoke reactance, and squelch the young person's hopes and dreams for the future, even if they are not realistic from your point of view.

PRACTITIONER: To help me understand more about you, I am wondering if you are willing to share how you see things in your future? What do you imagine life will be like, say 5 years from now?

YOUNG PERSON: Well, I want to work with younger kids like in a school or camp.

PRACTITIONER: You are interested in working with children. You said you like to have fun, so I bet you would be good at it. How does smoking marijuana fit with this goal?

YOUNG PERSON: Well, I guess if I have that type of job, I will only be able to smoke after work. (Change Talk)

PRACTITIONER: So one place you might consider a change is to cut back to only smoking at night.

By exploring the discrepancy between current behaviors and goals, the practitioner is guiding the youth to consider harm reduction (decreasing all day smoking to only smoking at night).

Tip for Imagining Questions: Try an Activity

Some young people may prefer to imagine beyond the use of verbal communications. For example, with permission, you can have the young person draw representations of "looking forward" and "looking back," or act out scenes showing "the best case scenario if I change" and "worst case scenario if I don't change." These activities can take on a playful or serious tone, depending on the young person's preferences.

Values Questions

Similar to looking forward and contrasting the young person's hopes and dreams with his or her current behavior, exploring incongruities between the young person's values with current behavior can elicit change talk (see Chapter 3 for further discussion of the rationale for developing discrepancy). By actively listening with OARS, you may already have clues to values that you can clarify with reflections, "It is really important to you to be independent." You may now follow with a comment to develop discrepancy, "I wonder how taking care of your health might fit with this value of being independent." The young person may then explain, "When I get sick, I have to rely on other people more." The desire to be an adult or to be treated as an older person can often be a powerful motivator for the young person, especially when the consequences of the current behavior result in being treated less like an adult (e.g., being "forced" to come to treatment, being placed in juvenile detention). A double-sided reflection can allow you to highlight the discrepancies in one succinct statement, a strategy often useful with young persons who prefer brief feedback (i.e., "On the one hand you value your independence, and on the other hand, your drug use has made you dependent on your dealer").

If the young person's values are not clear, you can ask pointed questions, such as "What things are important to you right now?" Inquiring about the characteristics of people who are important to the young person, or discussing positive attributes of a friend or boyfriend/girlfriend can also facilitate clarification of these issues.

PRACTITIONER: If it's OK with you to discuss, I'm wondering what are some things you like about your boyfriend?

YOUNG PERSON: Well, he is really nice, and he loves animals.

PRACTITIONER: Kindness is something you value.

Tip for Values Questions: Discuss the Balance between Short-Term Needs and Long-Term Values/Goals

It is important to express empathy around short-term needs (managing stress), which may be in conflict with long-term values and goals (graduating from high school, maintaining employment). You may even demonstrate this discrepancy with empathy, "It must be hard knowing that eating sugary foods satisfies your hunger, but yet can mess up your diabetes in the long run." You can then elicit the young person's ideas for change, "I wonder if there are foods that might meet both these needs—managing hunger and keeping your blood sugar under control?"

You can also discuss the effects of unsuccessful change attempts (actual or hypothetical) and how these may be related to important, but often neglected values. For example, in the case of Jenny struggling with weight, the practitioner explores how past attempts to follow a diet diverged from her value of having fun with friends (e.g., avoiding restaurants where friends hang out). Addressing this value in alternate ways may promote change.

PRACTITIONER: You mentioned having fun is really important to you. I am wondering if one reason you have not been able to follow a diet in the past is because it messed up your fun. (Reflection of Value)

JENNY: Yeah. I started to stay home more because I was trying to follow a meal plan. I would not go out with friends because I was afraid to eat at restaurants.

PRACTITIONER: It makes sense this did not work because you were not following what is really important to you, having fun with friends. I wonder if there is a meal plan that would allow you to go out with friends and go to restaurants. (Action Reflection)

JENNY: If there was, I bet I could follow it a lot better. (Change Talk)

Tip for Values Questions: Try an Experiential Activity to Elicit Values

The Values Card Sort, originally developed for MI by Sanchez (2001), has been effectively utilized in MI with young people (Resnicow et al., 2002). In this activity, after seeking permission from the young person, you provide a stack of cards with a value printed on each, along with an extra blank card so that a value can be added if your list does not include it. Next, you ask him or her to sort the cards into two piles, one for the more important and the other for the less important values. From the important value pile, he or she chooses the "top three values" that matter most to him or her. You then can ask open-ended questions regarding how the chosen values correspond with how the young person is currently living his or her life, paying particular attention to any discrepancies between the value and the problematic behavior (i.e., valuing health but smoking a pack of cigarettes a day). Open-ended questions can focus on elaboration about the value's personal meaning (i.e., "What does health mean to you?") and exploring areas where behavior does and does not correspond with the value (i.e., smoking cigarettes and health). It is critical that you incorporate reflections after each answer and before asking additional questions, particularly reflections that reinforce the change talk in the response.

Questions About Personal Strengths

There are several types of questions that you can use to support the young person's self-efficacy. You can encourage stories regarding past change successes related either directly to the target behavior or to other difficult changes. For example, "You mentioned you managed to keep the job at the gas station even though nobody helped you with transportation. How did you overcome this challenge?" Similarly, you can inquire about successfully accomplished goals from the past, personal strengths, or social supports available to help with overcoming challenges (e.g., "Who helped you? What are the things you did that made a difference?").

For the young person who does not easily identify personal strengths, you can explore what other people (friends, family) say about their strengths or good qualities. An Affirmation Card Sort activity may also help the young person identify these strengths. Akin to the Values Clarification exercise, the young person is first asked to choose qualities he or she possesses (e.g., thoughtful, kind, strong) from a list or stack of cards. You then follow up with similar questions about how these qualities are currently evident in the young person's life, in relation to both past successes and possible behavior change options. For example, "You mentioned you've always been a strong person. How might being a strong person help you if you decided to do something about your pot smoking?"

During this activity (and with all MI), you should convey your own hope and optimism regarding the young person's ability to change, as long at it is truly consistent with your belief. Research suggests that therapist optimism is a common factor evident in positive therapeutic outcomes (Lambert & Barley, 2001). For example, in the case of Jenny, the practitioner might comment, "You have been really persistent in trying to lose weight even though it has been so hard. I believe this persistence can really pay off once we can find the right strategy to help you lose weight."

ADDITIONAL STRATEGIES TO ELICIT CHANGE TALK

Rulers

Rulers are often incorporated into MI interventions (Miller & Rollnick, 2002). After asking permission, you describe or show a picture of the "ruler," with anchors of 1 as the lowest and 10 as the highest. You then ask the young person to rate on the ruler scale, from 1 to 10, "How important is it to you to change (problematic behavior)?" It is helpful to normalize the point scale. For example, "Some young people feel quitting smoking is not at all important and would rate a 1. Other youth believe this is the most important thing and would rate a 10. Others might be in the middle like a 4, 5, or 6. Where are you at?"

After the young person chooses a number, for example, a 4, your first task is to reflect the response and provide a contextual meaning for the chosen value (i.e., "You are somewhere in the middle. Changing this behavior might be important but maybe isn't your top priority"). Second, you should ask about why the young person did not choose a lower number (i.e., "Tell me why are you are a 4 and not a 1 or a 2"). By inquiring about lower numbers, you increase the likelihood that the young person will respond with change talk. That is, you are guiding him or her to defend a position in favor of change, rather than argue against it. For example, "Well, I know eventually I have to stop smoking, but I am not sure I want to right now." However, if you had asked a similarly phrased question, "Why were you a 4 and not a higher number?" you would have guided the young person to argue for reasons against change (e.g., "I really like smoking and it helps me to relax"). These slight shifts in your communication provide a critical distinction and tool for eliciting change talk instead of encouraging sustain talk. Note that if the person responds that they are a 1 on the ruler, this is a clue for you to return to strategies to respond to sustain talk (Chapter 5).

Tip for Rulers: Try the Ruler for Different Types of Change Talk

The ruler strategy may be used for other types of change talk, particularly ability (recall that readiness to change is a function of importance and ability). In a confidence ruler, the young person rates confidence in his or her ability to change on a 10-point scale. You might respond, "You say you are a 7. Though you are not 100% sure, you are pretty confident you could do this if you wanted to. Why are you a 7 and not a lower number?" Similar to the readiness ruler, exploring confidence with the scale elicits change talk, with the focus on personal abilities to change. Another possibility to promote engagement in treatment is to ask the young persons to rate how they feel about coming treatment (e.g., how much they want to come, how important it is to come, how confident they feel in being able to work with you). When you ask why the young person chose that number and not a lower number, you elicit reasons to engage in treatment!

Tip for Rulers: Try Asking What It Would Take to Get to a Higher Number

The question, "What would it take to get to a higher number?" also elicits change talk by requiring the young person to think about making a change without having to commit yet.

> PRACTITIONER: You said you were about a 5 in how ready you are to start exercising. Sort of ready but you're not sure. What would it take for you to be a higher number?
>
> JENNY: I guess if I could find something I like, I might be higher. I hated everything I've tried so far.
>
> PRACTITIONER: So if you found something you liked, you might consider exercising. You mentioned you used to dance, how do you feel about dancing now?

Personalized Feedback

There is some evidence to suggest that brief MI with young people that included feedback of assessment results had stronger effects on behavior change than brief MI without feedback (Walters, Vader, Harris, Field, & Jouriles, 2009). Personalized feedback involves presenting factual information about the young person's specific experiences with the target behavior, with the goals of increasing concern and developing discrepancy between the target behavior and the young person's goals/values. The information comes either from objective assessments (e.g., lab results, urine screens) or from the young person's own self-report rather than from the subjective reports of others. Utilizing the elicit–provide–elicit approach (EPE, described in Chapter 2), you will provide only facts, without judgment or your analysis of the results. Recall that interpretation of feedback is the young person's task, not yours.

> PRACTITIONER: What would you like to know about the questionnaires you completed?
>
> YOUNG PERSON: I was wondering what it was all about. I really don't drink that much.
>
> PRACTITIONER: Based on your report, if you add up the days you drank, you said you drank 20 out of the last 30 days for a total of 100 drinks. How does that fit with your thoughts about your drinking?

YOUNG PERSON: Well, I guess I did not realize I was drinking that much almost every day.

PRACTITIONER: You are wondering if you are drinking more than you realized.

YOUNG PERSON: Yeah, I'm OK with drinking, but I don't want to be a daily drinker. (Change Talk)

PRACTITIONER: Being a daily drinker does not fit with who you want to be. (Reflection of Discrepancy)

Personalized feedback simply summarizes the person's assessment results. In contrast, *normative* feedback facilitates the young person's comparison of him- or herself with similar others using population data (i.e., age, gender, race, etc.). For example, "You reported drinking about 20 drinks per week. Would you be interested in knowing how your use compares with others your age? This study here shows that young men ages 16–18 drink an average of 5 drinks per week." In providing information, some young persons may respond better to visual presentation (see Chapter 9), and the use of relevant norms specific to the young person (race, gender, age, geographic region) is key. If information is not available or is not specific to the young person, it is better to present personalized feedback instead. For example, young persons with HIV may not pay attention to normative substance abuse data from young people without HIV.

Some young people may reject being presented with normative data, as they may perceive themselves to be different from the norm, do not consider the behavior as a problem, and/or are not ready to make any changes. For example, "These data are old; everybody I know drinks as much as me." The young person may even question results from the objective assessment or the self-report questionnaires (i.e., "This can't be right, these questions are stupid anyway"). As with all forms of sustain talk, you can roll with these statements and further explore how the adolescent interprets their problematic behavior. For example, "OK, so as you see it, the assessment was not right. How much do you think you have been drinking, and what do you make of it?" In this way, you emphasize your respect for the young person's point of view while continuing to implement other, more relevant strategies.

SUMMARY

Do not worry about memorizing types of change talk. Recognizing change talk and selectively reinforcing it with OARS is the first step toward effecting a goal-directed interaction. We have presented several specific strategies to elicit change talk if it does not spontaneously emerge in the course of an OARS discussion. As throughout this guide, consider the strategies as a menu of options for you to choose from, and do not feel pressured to try all of them. The key is to consider trying the goal-oriented components of MI while maintaining the person-centered stance. With the young person, you must always be on the lookout for bumps in the road, as resistance may arise at any time. Which strategies to elicit change talk do you think fit with your personal style and expression of MI spirit?

SUMMARY: MI DOS AND DON'TS— RECOGNIZING AND REINFORCING CHANGE TALK

What to do	What not to do
Recognize change talk, regardless of type, and reinforce with OARS.	Miss opportunities to reinforce change talk, but avoid being too enthusiastic or too specific in asking for elaboration about change before the young person is committed to change.
Reflect when in doubt about how to respond.	Get lost in the journey of change or fall into the problem-solving trap.
Use open-ended questions that elicit change talk, not sustain talk.	Use closed-ended questions or interrogate with a series of questions.
Remember to balance questions with reflections.	Interrogate with a series of questions.
Try ruler exercises with questions to elicit change talk.	Ask for sustain talk using rulers (e.g., "Why are you that number and not a higher number?").
Use elicit–provide–elicit when giving personalized feedback.	Defend the "truth" of the data or dump information that is not relevant to the young person.
Elicit the relationship of feedback information to values and goals.	Insist on your own interpretation of the data.

CHAPTER 7

Commitment

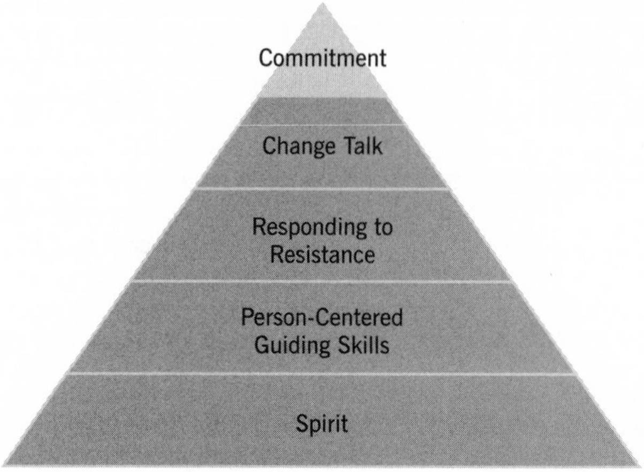
Commitment
Change Talk
Responding to Resistance
Person-Centered Guiding Skills
Spirit

> And what looks grand and remote so long as our words are still reaching out towards it from a long way off, later, once it has entered the sphere of our everyday activities, becomes quite simple and loses all its disturbing qualities.
>
> —ROBERT MUSIL, *Young Torless*

MI interventions support young people in making positive changes consistent with their personal values and goals. So far, we have focused on building motivation for change. In the next phase of the motivational interview, you will guide the young person to develop a plan for change and collaboratively consolidate commitment for change. This chapter focuses on two key questions you will face in facilitating this next phase of the conversation of change. First, how do you know when you have fully explored motivation for change and are ready to move to the specifics of a plan for change? Second, how do you consolidate commitment to a change plan?

MOVING TO THE NEXT PHASE
OF THE MOTIVATIONAL INTERVIEW

Listen for Change Talk of Increasing Strength

The best way to consider when to move to the next phase is to listen to the young person. As described in previous tasks, you listen for change talk and for sustain talk. First, you must focus your attention on the frequency and intensity of change talk. You should be hearing commitment language of increasing strength before moving on to a specific plan for change (see Table 7.1). The strongest change talk is commitment language. Examples include *"I am ready* to lose weight," *"I am willing* to cut back on my drinking," *"I will consider* taking my medication." Even stronger is commitment to a specific action, with stems such as "I will . . .," "I am going to . . .," and "I swear. . . ." In the case of Jenny, "I will check in with my mom in the evening and do the food log if she leaves me alone the rest of the day." Of course, you reinforce any commitment language with OARS, as these statements are the pearls in the ocean of change talk.

A key difference between MI and more directive approaches is that an MI practitioner waits for commitment language before developing a plan for change, whereas a more directive practitioner quickly moves to change plans or problem solving early in the encounter. For example, if the young

TABLE 7.1. Strength of Commitment Language (from Moyers's MISC manual)

1	2	3	4	5
"I mean to"	"I favor"	"I look	"I am devoted	"I guarantee"
"I foresee"	"I endorse"	forward to"	to"	"I will"
"I envisage"	"I believe"	"I consent to"	"I pledge to"	"I promise"
"I assume"	"I accept"	"I plan to"	"I agree to"	"I vow"
"I bet"	"I volunteer"	"I resolve to"	"I am prepared	"I shall"
"I hope to"	"I aim"	"I expect to"	to"	"I give my word"
"I will risk"	"I aspire"	"I concede to"	"I intend to"	"I assure"
"I will try"	"I propose"	"I declare my	"I am ready	"I dedicate
"I think I will"	"I am	intention to"	to"	myself"
"I suppose I	predisposed"			"I know"
will"	"I anticipate"			
"I imagine I	"I predict"			
will"	"I presume"			
"I suspect I				
will"				
"I contemplate"				
"I guess I will"				
"I wager"				
"I will see				
(about)"				

Note. From Miller, Moyers, Ernst, and Amrhein (2003). Reprinted with permission from the authors.

A key difference between MI and more directive approaches is that an MI practitioner waits for commitment language before developing a plan for change, whereas a more directive practitioner quickly moves to change plans or problem solving early in the encounter.

person is making statements such as "I going to do something about this problem," or "This is what I know I can do," this suggests that the young person is ready to make a plan for change. Statements such as "I think I might try" suggest continued ambivalence worthy of further exploration before moving to a specific change plan.

Listen for Diminishing Sustain Talk

Sustain talk should be diminishing (though it may not disappear!) with the increase in change talk and commitment language. Sustain talk may reemerge when discussing the specifics of a plan for change. We have learned that, especially with young people, backtracking to sustain talk happens often in the face of commitment! In the face of continued sustain talk, any efforts you make to guide the person to plan for change will be futile. Instead, your task at this time involves backing up the conversation, rolling with resistance, and further exploring ambivalence. Perhaps redefining the goal may be necessary (e.g., eating more fruits and vegetables instead of cutting calories). However, it is important to point out that ambivalence does not have to be completely resolved before moving along in discussing a change plan. For example, some behaviors are not intrinsically pleasurable (i.e., coming home at curfew) and may always elicit feelings of ambivalence ("I hate this, but I'll be home on time"). What matters is that the young person expresses change talk that is increasing in strength to the point where commitment emerges. You can reflect that ongoing ambivalence is a natural part of the journey of change. In our case of Jenny, sustain talk remerges when she begins to make a commitment to following a new eating plan. Of course if sustain talk continues, you may need to revert to other MI skills.

> JENNY: I know I have to lose weight so that I can have less knee pain but I can't stand feeling hungry! (Change Talk Followed by Sustain Talk)
>
> PRACTITIONER: You really want to make this change, and it will be easier if you can find some things to try when you feel hungry. (Action Reflection to Pave the Way toward a Change Plan)

In this next example, the practitioner empathically reflects the difficulty of having diabetes but does not stray from reinforcing commitment language and moving toward a plan for change.

YOUNG PERSON: I must start taking insulin to stay out of the hospital, but I still hate taking these shots.

PRACTITIONER: You seem really committed to making this change for your health, and of course you will never enjoy injecting yourself. What ideas do you have that might help make it easier? (Reflection and Question for Change Plan)

TRANSITIONING TO THE PLANNING PHASE: TESTING THE WATER

Use a summary to transition to the next phase of the interview, developing a plan for change. This summary first synthesizes the ambivalence discussions, highlights the strength of the commitment to change, and ends with a key question. In the case of Jenny, the practitioner summarizes, "We have talked about a lot of different things about eating. You said you don't think you have a problem with your eating, but you do want to lose weight. You don't want to go on a diet, but you are interested in eating healthier. So what do you think you'll do next?" Key questions are focused on guiding the young person to explore how he or she might go about change and engage in next steps (see Table 7.2). In addition, key questions allow you to test the water when you are unsure whether it is the appropriate time to transition and begin discussing a change plan.

If the young person's response to the key question is reminiscent of sustain talk (i.e., "I'd like to but . . ."), it may be premature to move to a plan focusing on behavior change. Alternatively, some remaining ambivalence should be expected, and your main task at this stage is to reflect it. Of course, if sustain talk continues, you may need to revert to earlier MI skills. To continue the example above, the practitioner asked a key question, "What do you think you will do?" and Jenny responds with some ambivalence related to her ability to make a change.

TABLE 7.2. Key Questions to Evoke Change Planning

"What else might you do?"

"How do you foresee yourself making these changes?"

"Why else do you think you could succeed?"

"What are some other reasons you think now is the time to make these changes?"

"What are your plans for the next week?"

JENNY: Well, I am not sure how to get started.

PRACTITIONER: So you are thinking about making a change in your eating, but you are not sure how to begin. Some people find it helpful to work out a plan for making a change. If you are interested, we can talk about some options and write down the steps you might want to take. (Reflection and Elicit Permission for Change Plan)

Tip for Transitioning to the Planning Phase: Consider Postponing Change Plans in the Face of High Emotional Intensity

Young people may express varying degrees of emotional intensity based on internal processes (e.g., hormones) and external stimuli (e.g., friends, family). For example, a young person may be leading up to a change plan, as demonstrated by increasing commitment language and decreasing sustain talk across sessions. However, if he or she has an argument with a parent or a breakup with a boyfriend/girlfriend right before the session, it may be difficult to engage the young person in the planning process at this time. The situation evoking this intensity may be tied to reasons for change, but the rational change planning process may best be put on hold until the young person feels less charged in the moment.

DEVELOPING A PLAN

In guiding young persons to plan for change, it is important that you not only understand their intention and motivation, but also help them be concrete and specific about what they will change and how they will implement the plan (Gollwitzer, 1999). In MI, this is accomplished via the formation of a change plan, a map for change where the young person draws in as much detail as possible to diminish the likelihood of getting lost.

Components of the Change Plan

The components include setting a goal, delineating steps to reach that goal, reviewing reasons to reach the goal, identifying potential barriers, and deciding on what to do to overcome barriers.

We next turn to the specific components of the change plan, including sample questions to elicit specificity, and issues to consider during this discussion (see Table 7.3). The components include setting a goal, delineating steps to reach that goal, reviewing reasons to reach the goal, identifying potential barriers, and

TABLE 7.3. Components of a Change Plan

Change plan component	Examples	Issues to consider
Set a goal.	• "What, if anything, would you like to work on for next time?" • "Based on what we talked about today, what would you consider to be a personal goal?"	• Are goals reasonable, attainable, and consistent with motivation to change? • Have you discussed intermediary goals, such as thinking about behavior change or issues of attendance and participation during the encounter?
Decide on steps to take to reach the goal.	• "What steps do you need to take to get started?" • "When would be a good time to start?"	• Are you falling into the expert trap? • Have you slipped into a paternalistic mode and "warned" the young person about issues he or she should be discussing? • Are you more enthusiastic about change than the young person?

deciding on what to do to overcome barriers. After these steps are completed, you affirm the young person's ideas, boost self-efficacy with statements of hope and optimism, and summarize.

Although we present the change plan process in a logical and stepwise manner, not all steps will necessarily be completed in any one encounter, and the order is flexible. Much akin to the skill of learning a new musical instrument, you should not expect the young person to be able to play a concerto or be able to engage in an entirely novel repertoire of behaviors after completing one single change plan. However, a guiding style will allow you to collaboratively map out possible paths toward change, consistently using person-centered counseling skills in an autonomy-supporting environment. Again, motivation to change is not static. The reemergence of sustain talk is common, especially in the face of practitioner enthusiasm for change and goal setting beyond the person's readiness. Thus, you should continue to balance all questions with reflections and continue to proceed cautiously, emphasizing personal choice and responsibility.

Here is an appropriate time to offer information or advice (with permission) in a guiding style as young people may not independently have all the necessary resources to fully consider all their options for a realistic change plan. We find the elicit–provide–elicit strategy (see Chapter 2) useful for offering a menu of options for change. For example, in the case of Jenny, the practitioner might begin, "If you're interested, I can share some things other teens have tried." With Jenny's permission, "Some people have started by adding a new fruit each week, others have tried to switch out Coke for water, and others have decided to limit the number of times they eat fast food in a week. What ideas do you have about specific steps to get started?" If the young person chooses one of the options you suggested, highlighting the fact that it was his or her choice is key to fostering individual autonomy. Emphasizing the word "you" is helpful. "So Jenny, you want to start by drinking water instead of coke. What meal would you like to start with for now?"

Tip for Change Plans: Increase Specificity of the Change Plan

In the above scenario, the practitioner also asks for more specificity to consolidate commitment, as the likelihood of success increases when you guide the young person to make a concrete and doable plan. The discussion of potential behaviors the young person will perform in the face of particular barriers to the goal will also consolidate commitment. Do not hesitate to use your expertise (with permission) and offer options for these potential barriers once you have elicited all barriers from the young person, as doing so increases the specificity of the plan. One example of offering options involves use of an omission reflection (Chapter 4). For example, "You did not mention anything that might get in the way of sticking to your food plan. Some kids have trouble when they are with their friends or when they are stressed out. What have you thought might get in the way?"

Tip for Change Plans: Goals Should Be Consistent with Length of Intervention

Some behavior change goals require many steps and many barriers to overcome (e.g., weight loss). Others may be reasonable in a very brief intervention (e.g., join a gym). For broad behavior change goals, consider more intensive treatments (see Chapter 7) and consider guiding the young person to develop a change plan around engaging in those treatments (either with you or with another practitioner).

Verbal and Written Change Plans

A change plan can be prepared verbally or via written methods. Table 7.3 details the pros and cons of each method. We suggest that your choice of strategy be based on the young person's individual needs. Similarly, we recommend that you not limit yourself to one modality or the other (even during the context of one encounter), as both lead to the same goal of collaborating with the young person about a specific change plan. In short, your overall mission is to be flexible, incorporating whichever strategy (or combination of strategies) the young person best responds to while discussing the change plan.

Change Plans for Young People Not Yet Ready to Change

You may find you are a better guide when you utilize the change plan process at the end of each session even when the young person is not yet ready to make major changes in behavior. In this case, options include making a small change (e.g., cut back one cigarette a day), thinking about change (e.g., talk to a friend, search information on the Internet), or coming back for another session with you or someone else. However, it is important that you always offer the young person the option of skipping the change plan discussion in these cases. It is especially important to tread carefully in this water, as you may unintentionally create a situation that elicits a decrease in the young person's motivation by asking for change when he or she is clearly not ready. Incorporating reflective statements to demonstrate your understanding of the young person's continued ambivalence can help to guard against this situation.

Note the balancing of reflections and questions in this dialogue.

PRACTITIONER: We are about finished with our time today, and this is when you might consider setting a goal for yourself. I understand you are not yet ready to make a change. If it's OK with you, we can set a goal around something you are ready to do. What do you think about that? (Elicit Permission)

YOUNG PERSON: I am not sure what you mean because I am not going to quit drinking.

PRACTITIONER: Well, your goal could be about another area of your life like school or friends, or to think about our discussion today, or maybe just to come back next time. (Provide) What do you think? (Elicit Response)

YOUNG PERSON: I guess my goal could be to come back next week to get my parents off my back.

PRACTITIONER: So you would want to come back next week. (Reflection) What would it take to get you here? (Open-Ended Question)

YOUNG PERSON: Well, we have to set up a time that will work for me, and I have to figure out a way to get here.

PRACTITIONER: That's great you have some thoughts about how to reach your goal. (Affirmation) If we set up a time that works for you, how will you get here? (Elaboration)

YOUNG PERSON: I guess I can ask my parents or take the bus.

PRACTITIONER: So you have some transportation options. (Reflection) What might get in the way? (Open-Ended Question)

YOUNG PERSON: If I am hanging out with my friends, I won't want to come. Or if I have a fight with my parents, I may want to skip it to make them mad.

PRACTITIONER: If you are with your friends or get mad at your parents, you might not feel like coming. (Reflection) How could you overcome these barriers to reach your goal of attending next week? (Open-Ended Question)

YOUNG PERSON: I am not sure. I guess I could make sure I don't see my friends before our meeting and maybe not my parents either. Maybe I should try to come right after school is out.

ADDITIONAL STRATEGIES TO CONSOLIDATE COMMITMENT

As noted earlier, the change planning process itself, by articulating specific plans for change, helps to consolidate the young person's commitment. OARS may also be tailored for this phase. When summarizing the change plan, include reflections of previous change talk (i.e., "As you said, now is probably the best time to do something about your problem"). Open-ended questions that directly elicit commitment language (see Chapter 6) are also fruitful (e.g., "Why do you feel this is something you must do?" "Why do you feel now is the time for a change?"). As described in Chapter 6, always reinforce the commitment language you elicit with these questions with OARS. Other strategies used in earlier stages of the motivational interview may also be adapted at this time. For example, a hybrid of the ruler strategy (see Chapter 5) without use of a 1–10 scale (as commitment should not be a 1 or 2 at this stage) can be effective in eliciting commitment.

PRACTITIONER: So you have a lot of ideas about how to make this happen. How sure are you that you are going to follow through with this plan? Sort of sure, very sure, or totally sure?

YOUNG PERSON: I am pretty sure I will do it.

PRACTITIONER: What makes you pretty sure versus something less?

YOUNG PERSON: Well, I know I will just get worse if I don't, and I really want a better future for myself than my parents think I do.

PRACTITIONER: So this plan is something you are pretty sure you will follow through on because YOU think it is important for your future. It's not about what your parents think. What would it take for you to be more sure?

Following up with a question like this can elicit other potential barriers for discussion. Another way to consolidate commitment is to visualize the change that will occur. In the previous example, "What does this future look like?" This can be done verbally, visually (e.g., drawing), or playfully (e.g., pretend role-play).

FOLLOW-UP VISITS

Although a change plan can occur at any time during your first or follow-up visit with the young person, we find the change plan process useful to end each session consistent with the goal-oriented component of MI. Follow-up sessions may focus on a review of the initial change plan and then a refinement or revision. Change is a journey that one travels throughout the lifespan, and the old notion of two steps forward and one step back often prevails. Any progress the young person makes toward healthy behavior change or goal achievement, however miniscule it may appear to you, represents movement in a positive direction. It is important that you reflect this and provide affirmation while avoiding overenthusiasm. It is especially important to respond to difficulties completing the change plan with empathy and a nonjudgmental stance. Based on the level of change talk and sustain talk that arises in this discussion, you may return to an earlier phase of MI or discuss a revision or elaboration of the change plan. Most importantly, we emphasize that MI spirit and skills, along with a developmental perspective, will allow you to guide the young persons to maximize their potential along the path of their choice.

SUMMARY

Guiding the young person to develop a change plan consistent with his or her personal goals and consolidating commitment to that plan is the second phase of MI. We have discussed how to recognize when to move into this phase based on the strength of change talk and commitment language, as well as reductions in sustain talk. We have also noted that the reemergence of ambivalence is common, but should not derail the change plan process if it is fleeting. Increasing specificity of the change plan, as well as identifying behaviors to overcome barriers, will increase its chance of success. The key to developing a change plan in the spirit of MI is balance: balance of eliciting the young person's ideas with offering information or advice; balance of your use of questions and reflections; and balance of your expressions of optimism and hope with the development of realistic and attainable goals. What components of balance do you plan to integrate when you develop treatment plans with young people?

SUMMARY: MI DOS AND DON'TS– CONSOLIDATING COMMITMENT

What to do	What not to do
Assess readiness to complete a change plan based on increasing strength of change talk and response to key questions.	Move to a plan for behavior change if change talk is weak or significant sustain talk is still present. Consider a change plan around continuing the discussion instead.
Evoke the young person's ideas for change and offer a menu of options with permission.	Fall into the expert trap by offering what you think is best without permission.
Elicit barriers to change and guide the young person to make "if–then" plans.	Be afraid to bring up potential obstacles (with permission).
Ask open-ended questions to elicit commitment to the change plan.	Ignore remaining ambivalence (but don't let it derail you if it is fleeting).
Express hope and optimism about the young person's ideas and abilities.	Be overly enthusiastic about specific changes in behavior.

CHAPTER 8

❋　　❋　　❋　　❋

Integrating Motivational Interviewing into Your Practice

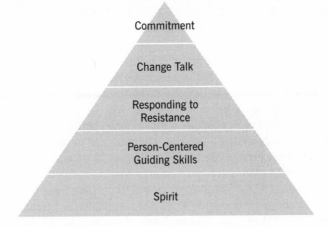

Commitment

Change Talk

Responding to Resistance

Person-Centered Guiding Skills

Spirit

Within a change process is a period of not having the old way of thinking, while not yet integrating the new way of thinking, which is the chaos of creativity at an important juncture.
—JAN SHEPPARD

Integrating MI into your own practice and setting defines the final stage in learning MI. We believe the spirit of MI and person-centered communication skills should characterize interactions with all patients. However, MI interventions are most appropriate for those ambivalent about change, as the exploration of ambivalence may be counterproductive for those ready to change. Although the spirit of MI is a natural therapeutic stance, and MI can be a platform for all interventions or session activities (Arkowitz & Westra, 2004), what is most important is that you are appropriately choosing to use MI with your clients when the core issue involves motivation to change. We next turn to discussing the integration of MI into brief interventions as well as longer treatments.

INTEGRATION OF MI IN BRIEF INTERVENTION SETTINGS

MI is often integrated in settings where a single session is offered. The length of the session can range from a brief 10- to 15-minute interaction (e.g., medical consultation, community outreach) to a longer visit (e.g., intake interview, therapy session). For example, MI has been used with young people in a brief interaction by outreach workers to promote HIV counseling and testing (see Chapter 12) or in an emergency room to encourage reduction in alcohol consumption (see Chapter 9). MI may also be offered as a pretreatment—a prelude to increase motivation to engage in a longer-term treatment. In these approaches, MI may be provided by different practitioners and sometimes by different agencies than those offering the more intensive treatment. Examples include MI by an intake worker to increase motivation for inpatient substance abuse treatment, MI by an inpatient mental health provider to increase motivation to follow up with outpatient care, or MI to promote engagement in a subsequent group intervention.

Several skills described in earlier chapters are particularly useful for brief interventions. First, it is critical to identify a specific target behavior because you typically will not have enough time to focus on multiple areas of behavior change in a brief intervention. Often, the target behavior is set by the constraints of the system (e.g., MI to engage in further substance abuse treatment, MI to encourage counseling and testing). However, within these constraints, there should still be options from which the young person can choose his or her desired focus for the session. For example, if substance use is the target, the young person may choose to focus on a particular substance or choose between a moderation focus and an abstinence focus. As always, there should be an option to address other issues that may be more critical at that moment than the target behavior (e.g., problems with a girlfriend) that can be tied to the ultimate goal toward the end of the session (see Chapter 2). Beginning with agenda-setting strategies when your time is limited (see Chapter 3) can help to quickly identify the target behavior for the session.

> MI spirit suggests forgoing the traditional assessment process and diagnostic interview in favor of eliciting the young person's point of view using OARS.

MI spirit suggests forgoing the traditional assessment process and diagnostic interview in favor of eliciting the young person's point of view using OARS. If an assessment is required at the onset of treatment (as is common in many agencies), one option may be to first elicit the young person's point of view with active listening skills (OARS) and complete the paperwork based on the information you obtain. Another option may be to balance assessment questions with reflections and summaries.

In a brief session, agenda setting moves quickly into a brief discussion of the target behavior using OARS to build rapport, reinforce any change talk, and elicit change talk if not present. As the chapters in the next section of this book indicate, feedback is often used as a strategy in brief interventions to develop discrepancy between current behaviors and the young person's goals and values (see Chapter 6). Of course, with a young person you may find that almost the entire session is spent rolling with resistance and guiding the young person to even consider behavior change in follow-up sessions with you or another provider. Brief sessions often end with some form of a change plan. In brief interventions, it may be necessary to move into goal setting even if the young person is not ready to change. Chapter 6 describes ways to do this carefully without eliciting resistance.

INTEGRATING MI WITH OTHER TREATMENTS

MI provides the platform for a good therapy process regardless of the specific intervention framework you may be using. As David Olds has noted, MI is a powerful ingredient that fuels good practice. Of course you will want to add other ingredients either by following a recipe (e.g., a manualized treatment) or by adding a little bit of this and a little bit of that from whichever theoretical background you practice. The majority of studies demonstrating the efficacy of MI integrated with other behavior change methods for young people have focused on behavioral treatments (for review, see Erickson, Gerstle, Feldstein, 2005; Sindelar, Abrantes, Hart, Lewander, & Spirito, 2004; Suarez & Mullins, 2008). We next provide a summary and examples of applications for how we believe MI can be integrated within the two predominant behavioral modalities used with young populations, specifically, cognitive-behavioral interventions and extrinsic motivation approaches.

> MI provides the platform for a good therapy process regardless of the specific intervention framework you may be using.

Cognitive-Behavioral Treatments and MI

MI has most commonly been integrated with cognitive-behavioral treatments (CBT) (see the chapters in Part II for examples). CBT focuses on teaching the young person specific skills (i.e., coping, problem solving, assertiveness training, self-monitoring, and cognitive restructuring) and incorporates specific assignments to facilitate the acquisition and generalization of skills to the young person's natural environment. The underlying premise of CBT suggests that young persons have a skill deficit, and if they are taught and learn certain skills, they will then be able to improve functioning and experience less psychological distress.

Briefly, in CBT the practitioner determines which skills to target by completing a functional assessment of the antecedent interpersonal and environmental factors that promote or sustain the young person's problematic responses (including both intrusive cognitions and behaviors). This is done in an interview format (typically a series of questions). While the importance of collaboration about goals is an important component of any CBT, the emphasis on relationship factors is not a central focus for the practitioner. Rather, the emphasis is on the teaching and use of skills. CBT can be an important adjunct to MI, particularly in young people who may not have fully developed the skills necessary for behavior change. Indeed, when CBT is conducted without MI spirit and skills, there is a danger that the young person will not engage in the work necessary for skill attainment and perhaps will actively resist such change.

In CBT, you may use MI at the onset of treatment to elicit motivation for the skills training component of the intervention, and throughout the treatment to solidify commitment to therapy goals and completion of "homework." After the functional assessment, MI remains a platform for delivering the skills (see Table 8.1 for specific examples). MI is especially

TABLE 8.1. MI to Enhance Cognitive-Behavioral Treatments

CBT	MI plus CBT
Treatment begins with an overview and rationale for treatment followed by a functional assessment of the target behavior.	Treatment begins with eliciting the client's view (Chapter 3) and increasing motivation for change by eliciting and reinforcing change talk (Chapter 6).
Functional assessment is completed in an interview fashion (typically a series of questions).	The functional assessment is completed in the context of an OARS conversation and may also incorporate feedback from questionnaires (see Chapter 6).
Practitioner chooses skills modules based on functional assessment of triggers and consequences.	Practitioner elicits the young person's thoughts and ideas to manage triggers and guides the young person toward skills modules to meet the young person's goals in a change plan (Chapter 7).
Homework is assigned with a rationale provided by the practitioner.	Homework is suggested with permission to meet the young person's goals (elicit–provide–elicit; Chapter 3).

helpful to address resistance or ambivalence that arises during cognitive-behavioral skills training. For example, consider a young person who presents with a goal of reducing anxiety, but is avoidant of committing to difficult treatments, (i.e., exposure to feared stimuli or the initiation of psychotropic medications; see Chapter 14). At the onset of treatment, you might be able to reduce initial ambivalence to anxiety treatments with the use of MI skills. After eliciting and reinforcing change talk, the young person may agree to a change plan that includes further treatment. However, as is common in clinical practice, you may find after several visits that treatment tasks are not being accomplished (i.e., assigned homework for exposure or compliance with a medication regimen) or sustain talk reemerging (e.g., "I am not sure all this [exposure treatment] is worth it. It's too hard."). You may then switch to using MI skills such as rolling with resistance, exploring ambivalence with open-ended questions, eliciting and reinforcing change talk, and developing discrepancy between values/goals. When you again hear change talk of increasing strength and can reconsolidate commitment to the change plan, you may switch back to the more directive treatment.

Extrinsic Motivation Approaches and MI

Many treatments for young people include strategies to target extrinsic motivation. Examples include contingency management approaches (i.e., the young person receives monetary rewards or vouchers for abstinence to substance use), token economies (i.e., the young person earns points for compliance in inpatient or residential settings), and family behavior plans (i.e., the parent provides rewards or punishments for the adolescent's compliant or noncompliant behaviors). Contexts and treatment settings operating from an extrinsic motivational system often are limited in the amount of choice and decision-making responsibility afforded to the young person. These typically mandated situations can increase the young person's resistance to treatment. The integration of MI into these settings holds promise for improving engagement and personal responsibility.

Historically, extrinsic motivation and intrinsic motivation were thought to be polar opposites, with the former undermining the latter. However, Deci, Koestner, and Ryan's (1999) research suggests otherwise. That is, investigations about intrinsic and extrinsic motivation in young persons have shown them to be separate phenomena, and not inversely related (Lepper, Corpus, & Iyengar, 2005). Other researchers have pointed to the additive effect of intrinsic and extrinsic motivational approaches (i.e., targeting internal motivators, such as achievement of personal goals, and simultaneously using external motivators, such as offering monetary incentives for goal attainment).

Targeting both aspects of motivation may have a synergistic effect. You may tip the scale of ambivalence, even if temporarily, with an extrinsic reward, while simultaneously utilizing MI skills to promote the identification of internal reasons for doing the new behavior (Carroll et al., 2006; Vallerand, 1997). We now give several examples of specific skills needed to successfully integrate MI with extrinsic reinforcement approaches.

Proposing Rewards

When you offer extrinsic reinforcers (i.e., money or extra time to engage in planned activities, such as spending time with friends or playing video games) without offering choice in decisions (i.e., in a controlling manner), intrinsic motivation decreases (Deci & Ryan, 1985). In contrast, if you offer extrinsic motivators in a more pro-choice fashion (i.e., informationally), the target behavior is more likely to be internalized. We demonstrate this difference with two examples. Although both begin with a reflection, the first is a controlling approach while the second offers choice.

> CONTROLLING PRACTITIONER: So we've talked a lot about how you need to finish off your probation hours. If it's OK with you, next I need to review what I need you to do next.
>
> INFORMATIONAL PRACTITIONER: So we've talked a lot about finishing off your probation hours. If it's ok with you, I'd like to next talk about options to finish off your probation hours and how I support you in your choice.

Addressing Resistance to Extrinsic Motivation Approaches

Resistance is diminished when you implement extrinsic motivational approaches in the context of MI conversations that support autonomy and self-efficacy. Your use of OARS is important for decreasing the resistance common in traditional extrinsic reinforcement treatments, particularly those emphasizing consequences. In this way, MI not only promotes internal motivation, but also addresses the psychological reactance expected from the young person in contexts that restrict behavior and limit choices. You can use reflections to reiterate the reality of the situation while still demonstrating empathy and respect for the young person.

Examples

Reflection of feeling: "You are really frustrated you have to deal with this point system in order to be released from the hospital."

Double-sided reflection: "You are angry right now. You are getting consequences for being out late but part of you might also be glad to earn back privileges peacefully."

Reflection followed by a question: "You don't like to be told what to do, but you have to follow these rules to be released from probation. What thoughts do you have to make this easier?"

Action reflection: "If we can figure out how to get the probation officer off your back, life will be a whole lot easier."

Pros and cons: "What bothers you about this behavior plan? What are some good things that could happen if you follow it?"

MI to Elicit Change Talk in External Motivation Approaches

Strategies to elicit change talk and solidify commitment may also be utilized to build self-efficacy and promote intrinsic motivation in the context of extrinsic motivational treatments. Of course, these strategies are best utilized after responding to sustain talk and solidifying rapport.

Examples

Eliciting strengths: "You were able to complete your homework so that you didn't lose your Playstation. How were you able to manage this?"

Value–behavior discrepancy: "You completed 30 minutes of exercise so you could get your prize and you said that you felt stronger when you did it. How does that fit with what you said about being a strong, independent person?"

Looking forward: "I know that right now you are only doing this to get off probation. What would life be like if you continued this behavior change?"

SUMMARY

There are several ways to include MI in your repertoire of clinical interventions, ranging from using MI in brief settings to using it as a platform from which all other treatments are offered. How might you integrate MI with other clinical interventions you use with young people? We next turn to examples of MI for subpopulations of young persons with specific behavioral change issues. These chapters address interventions based solely on MI, as well as interventions combining MI with other approaches.

Summary MI Dos and Don'ts: Intgrating MI with Other Interventions

What to do	What not to do
Use MI to engage the young person in more intensive treatments.	Use MI to explore ambivalence when the young person is ready to change.
Return to goal-oriented MI skills when ambivalence arises during other treatments such as CBT.	Derail other treatments when ambivalence is present but fleeting (some ambivalence may always be present, particularly around unpleasant behaviors such as taking insulin or managing hunger).
Use MI spirit and person-centered communication as a platform for good practice in any treatment approach.	Use MI as a panacea for all problems.

PART II

✻   ✻   ✻

SIDE TRIPS

CHAPTER 9

✳   ✳   ✳   ✳

Alcohol Problems

Lynn Hernandez, Nancy Barnett, Holly Sindelar-Manning,
Thomas H. Chun, and Anthony Spirito

SCOPE OF THE PROBLEM

Alcohol use among youth is a significant public health concern. Over 39% of high school students report beginning alcohol use before age 13 (Johnston, O'Malley, Bachman, & Schulenberg, 2008). By the time young people reach the 12th grade, 55% report having been drunk and 25% report binge drinking (5+ drinks once or twice each weekend in the last 30 days; Johnston et al., 2008). Furthermore, less than half of high school seniors perceive harm in binge drinking once or twice each weekend (Johnston et al., 2008). While multiple pathways lead to alcohol use in young people, including developmentally normative experimentation (Schulenberg, Maggs, Steinman, & Zucker, 2001), Hawkins and colleagues (1997) found that early initiation of alcohol use increases the risk of developing alcohol-related problems and DSM-IV diagnoses during adulthood.

WHY MI?

There are several reasons why MI is a promising approach for young people with alcohol use problems. First, MI is most appropriate for individuals who have not yet reached the severe end of the spectrum of a specific health risk behavior. In general, young people, because of their relative youth, have not experienced the extent of physical and psychosocial consequences of drinking that many adults have experienced. Second, MI interventions are oriented toward reductions in alcohol-related behaviors (e.g., harm-reduction approaches), a goal that may be more realistic and attainable than long-term cessation/abstinence or avoidance of drinking. Third, adolescents rarely admit to or recognize alcohol use problems, and seldom seek treatment on their own. MI's use of behavioral change principles and motivational engagement strategies in a nonjudgmental and nonconfrontational style may be particularly useful for engaging young people who have little motivation to change. Last, MI's underlying assumption that self-change is the predominant pathway to making positive changes to drinking behaviors is concurrent with one of the primary developmental tasks during adolescence—self-development. Adolescents will be more convinced by arguments directing them toward change that they have thought of themselves. Therefore use of MI techniques (i.e., rolling with resistance and complex reflections) to elicit change talk makes this approach congruent with this particular developmental task.

MI *Spirit and Strategies*

The MI approach described here has been used with over 200 young people recruited from an Emergency Department where they received care for an alcohol-related injury (Monti et al., 1999; Spirito et al., 2004). The intervention consists of five components: introduction and engagement, exploration of motivation, enhancement of motivation, establishing a change plan, and enhancing self-efficacy.

Introduction and Engagement

The introduction provides the young person with an idea of the MI content and how the young person's time will be spent with the practitioner. We introduce the session as an opportunity for young persons to obtain information about their own pattern of drinking and to spend some time, if they are interested, talking about ways to avoid problems related to alcohol use. Practitioners emphasize that they will not tell the young person what to do; rather, it is up to the young person to make choices about drinking and about what he or she does when drinking. In the case where an alcohol-related event (such as medical treatment for intoxication or an alcohol-related injury) led to the MI, we review circumstances of this event, including how much the young person drank, who he or she was with, and what type of problem resulted.

The introduction also provides an opportunity to minimize defensiveness. Open-ended questions are used to enhance rapport and help the practitioner develop an understanding of the young person's recent drinking patterns and problems that developed. The practitioner should present as empathic, concerned, nonauthoritarian, and nonjudgmental, a style that is central to MI (see Chapter 3). It is important, for example, that you be respectful of the young person's experiences, and not make either disapproving or reassuring statements about the young person's behavior.

In our protocol, assessment measures serve as both outcome measures and as a means to personalize feedback. Assessments are administered after the MI program has been described to the young person. Assessments are chosen to provide young people with a perspective on how they compare to other young people and to give them information about the risks that may arise secondary to their alcohol use. In order to provide such "normative information," it is best to use measures that have both age and gender norms available.

Exploration of Motivation

Once the assessment is complete, you ask the young person what he or she likes and does not like about drinking. Open-ended questions and reflective listening statements are used to encourage the young persons to generate as many likes and dislikes as possible (i.e., pros and cons) and to talk about the effects of alcohol, positive and negative, that matter to them most. The young persons are also asked what they perceive might be positive about engaging in risky behaviors after drinking, as well as the worst things they could imagine happening if they did engage in these risky behaviors. Finally, they are asked to discuss parents' and friends' attitudes toward drinking and how those attitudes might affect their own drinking behaviors.

By the conclusion of this section of the MI session, you should have a fairly clear understanding of the young person's decisional balance with respect to drinking. The pros and cons are not used as a technique to manage resistance or to elicit change talk but to allow you and the young person to share her or his understanding of positive reinforcers for drinking that should be acknowledged—that is, the pros as well as the perceived cons that might function as reasons for reducing alcohol use. However, when you use complex reflections, particularly after the young person has stated the perceived cons to drinking (e.g., "The idea of being kicked off the football team really scares you"), you can elicit change talk during this exercise. This discussion also helps you to identify peer and parental influences on the drinking behavior, and the importance of these influences. You can then tailor the MI to these personalized pros and cons, while keeping in mind the young person's stage of readiness for changing his or her drinking behavior.

Enhancement of Motivation

This section of the MI is designed to increase young people's understanding of their patterns of alcohol use, provide information about indicators of problem drinking, and promote interest in making positive changes to hazardous drinking. This is done in three ways. First you provide personalized feedback from the assessment measures, including interpretation of the young person's scores compared to age and gender norms. Second, you offer information about alcohol and its effects, such as the effects of blood alcohol concentration levels on behavior, and alcohol's effects on driving skills. And third, you ask the young person to discuss how he or she imagines the future would be like if he or she were to change, or not change.

Personalized Feedback

The computer program we developed generates a printed personalized feedback sheet that summarizes information collected during the assessment. The feedback report uses age- and gender-based normative information to compare the young persons to their peers. Percentile ranks are provided for drinking frequency and quantity, frequency of five or more drinks on occasion, and alcohol-related problems affecting family, friends, and school. These data are presented in graphical form. Examples of physical and emotional dependence, including signs of tolerance and withdrawal, as well as the risk taking that occurs with alcohol use are provided. As in other parts of the interview, you make decisions about what aspects of the feedback on which to focus and what aspects to deemphasize. You ask young people what they were most surprised by in the feedback and what was of most concern to them. You help the young person interpret the personal meaning of the feedback. If a young person has an extreme profile, you can encourage her or him by being reminded that this negative information can improve with behavior change.

When relevant, information about blood alcohol level, rates of alcohol metabolization, and effects of alcohol on driving can be provided. In medical settings where young people are tested for their blood alcohol level, most are interested in their results and receptive to information about the effects of alcohol at different levels.

Envision the Future

You can further enhance motivation by asking young people to imagine the future both if their drinking were to remain the same and if it were to change. If it is established that a discrepancy exists between the young person's current drinking and his or her goals for the future, such a discrepancy may provide motivation and therefore should be explored by the clinician. For example, if a young person aspires to athletic achievement, the clinician might use a prompt such as "What would be different about your sports performance if you cut down on your drinking?" and "What would make it easier/harder to do this?" The use of double-sided reflections to point out the discrepancy can be useful in eliciting change talk from the young person.

Establish a Plan

Regardless of the treatment setting, or the focus or length of the MI, the young person should leave the session with a well-considered plan and make a commitment to that plan. Prior to discussing a plan, it is good for you to reassess the young person's interest in changing. Good open-ended questions to use include: "Where does this leave you now?" or "What if anything, would you like to change?"

If the young person is able to generate reasonable ways to reduce drinking, your main task is to help the young person examine barriers to implementation of the strategies. However, it is not unusual for young persons to be vague about what they would like to do differently, and you must help them develop a list of specific strategies. For example, a young person might say, "I won't drink so much." Your task in this case would be to help the young person specify a specific goal. Open-ended exploration questions, such as "Tell me how you might do that," can be useful. A more direct response might be, "We know that if you were to have no more than one drink an hour, your blood alcohol level would stay at a low level. What do you think about that for a goal?"

Developing a plan for those who are not interested in making any changes to their drinking is more challenging. In most cases there will be something the young person would like to avoid, such as getting hurt after drinking or getting into a car accident. In these situations, you can help develop a plan that focuses on harmful behaviors rather than alcohol consumption per se. Alternatively, young people may be interested in keeping track of their drinking or recording how much money they spend on alcohol over a defined period of time. In such cases, self-monitoring of drinks might be the behavior change goal. The goal, therefore, increasingly focuses on the young person's awareness of his or her drinking, which in turn may raise the young person's level of concern and lead to reduced consumption.

You should also provide a menu of specific and clear strategies to reach treatment goals. A variety of change strategies should be included to find something that the young person would be interested in trying. In this way, the young person is exposed to a larger number of possibilities and may actually select some things to do that may be more than what you expected. Nonetheless, whenever possible, young people should generate goals rather than have goals selected for them.

Goal setting is most successful when goals are personalized, concrete, and behavioral, and include a timeline. Young people should be encouraged to specify a time within the next few days when they will attempt one goal.

A copy of the list of goals and target dates should be provided at the end of the session.

Anticipate Barriers

While developing the behavior change plan, you should help the young person think about what might prove to be an obstacle in implementing the plan. For example, you could ask how the young person thinks his or her friends will react to the young person deciding not to drink one night on the weekend. Providing realistic hypothetical situations to discuss can make this part of the session more meaningful. Anticipating barriers in this fashion will help the young person identify challenges, and refine and change the plan if necessary to address these barriers. These steps can be a way to enhance the young person's self-efficacy.

Provide Advice

Giving advice about limiting drinking (i.e., the harm reduction approach) is especially controversial when working with minors. Clinicians are more likely to give advice when working with young people than adults. Advice is warranted when young people are not able to generate ideas very well, when they ask specifically for advice, or when they are not generating appropriate goals.

Enhance Self-Efficacy

If the young person makes a plan to change, it is critical that he or she feels positive about implementing this plan. Therefore, one of your primary tasks is to enhance the young person's sense that changes can be made effectively. Strategies to accomplish this goal might include reinforcing promising but realistic ideas; making supportive statements about the young person's strengths that will ensure success in carrying out the plan; and being optimistic about the young person's future once change is implemented.

RESEARCH IMPLICATIONS

Our research group has tested the version of MI described here in two studies. Monti and colleagues (1999) conducted a study evaluating the use of an MI intervention to reduce alcohol use and alcohol-related consequences among 18- and 19-year-old adolescents being treated in an urban hospital Emergency Department for an alcohol-related event. Ninety-four adolescents were randomly assigned to either the 40-minute MI intervention or the 5-minute "standard care" intervention (i.e., receiving a handout on avoiding drinking and driving and a substance treatment referral list). At the 6-month follow-up assessment, participants randomized to the MI condition showed lower alcohol-related problems than those in the standard care condition. Spirito and colleagues (2004) reported on the same brief MI intervention among 152 younger adolescents (13–17 years) involved in the Monti and colleagues study. Both conditions resulted in reduced quantity of drinking during the 12 months of follow-up, while alcohol-related negative consequences were relatively low and stayed low at follow-up in both groups. However, adolescents who screened positive for problematic alcohol use at the baseline assessment reported significantly more improvement on average number of drinking days per month and frequency of high-volume drinking if they received MI compared to standard care.

Further research should continue to examine the efficacy of MI among alcohol-using young people by comparing it to other active treatments designed to target alcohol use. Furthermore, research studies should be conducted in community sites, for example, in family court where young people are seen for minor alcohol-related offenses, in mental health clinics, and in pediatric practices, with particular attention paid to how pediatricians and care professionals can promote behavior change among young people. Finally, the use of MI with diverse ethnic/racial populations needs to be examined. Whether this therapeutic approach is effective with young people of diverse backgrounds or whether MI interventions need to be culturally adapted is unknown.

CHAPTER 10

❋　　❋　　❋　　❋

Marijuana Use

Denise Walker

SCOPE OF THE PROBLEM

Although marijuana use rates among adolescents and young adults have fluctuated over the past 30 years, marijuana continues to be the most prevalently used illicit substance (Johnston et al., 2008). For example, in 2007, the prevalence of 8th, 10th, and 12th graders reporting marijuana use was 14.2%, 31.0%, and 41.8%, respectively. *Daily* marijuana use was reported by 0.8% of 8th graders, 2.8% of 10th graders, and 5.1% of 12th graders. Young adults show the highest rates of use (SAMHSA, 2007). Among the multitude of adverse effects associated with these high rates of marijuana use by young people, the issue of greatest concern may be detriments to normal adolescent and young adult development, for example, poorer psychosocial outcomes such as lower educational attainment and greater use of other illicit drugs (Fergusson, Horwood, & Swain-Campbell, 2002).

A second concern pertains to the long-term impairing effects of use on cognition. Studies of adults using marijuana found that onset of use before 16 or 17 predicted poorer performance in tasks requiring focused attention (Ehrenreich et al., 1999) and lower verbal IQ (Pope et al., 2003). While these negative outcomes may well be caused by marijuana use, two alternative explanations can be considered. First, innate cognitive ability differences may exist between users and nonusers prior to initial use of marijuana. Second, those initiating marijuana use at younger ages may be more likely to avoid the academic learning experiences necessary for acquiring conventional cognitive skills.

A third issue pertains to the risk of increased mental health problems, particularly anxiety and depression. Onset of marijuana use prior to age 15, and frequent use at age 21, are associated with increased risks for experiencing both anxiety and depression in young adulthood (Hayatbakhsh et al., 2007). Finally, those young persons initiating use at very early ages, (i.e., prior to age 13, or using marijuana weekly or more often at midadolescence), present with an elevated risk of later dependence problems(Coffey, Carlin, Lynskey, Li, & Patton, 2003; Kokkevi, Nic Gabhainn, & Spyropoulou, 2006). Compared with adults, young persons with marijuana use qualify for a dependence diagnosis at lower frequencies and quantities of marijuana consumption (Chen, Kandel, & Davies, 1997).

Why MI?

Lack of motivation remains a key barrier in the treatment of marijuana abuse and dependence, and several clinical factors associated with adolescent marijuana use make MI a promising fit for intervention. First, young people often perceive marijuana as less harmful than other illicit drugs (Johnston et al., 2008), and MI offers a collaborative conversation for the young person to explore their perceptions without you having to take a paternalistic, "just say no," approach.

Second, young people often offer arguments supporting political and philosophical justification of marijuana use. For example, marijuana has been at the center of debates surrounding marijuana legalization and medicinal use, and common are statements such as "It's natural—so what's the big deal?" These arguments often add confusion to conversations about the negative consequences of the young person's use. With MI, you offer a nonjudgmental, nonconfrontational platform for the young person to explore the pros and cons of use for the young person's personal values and goals.

Third, few adolescents actually volunteer for treatment, and personal motivation to change use of marijuana is often rare. For example, 90% of adolescents meeting substance use disorder criteria are not enrolled in treatment (Titus at al., 1999). Referrals to treatment are typically prompted by the legal system, parents, or the school. For those actually presenting for treatment, only 20% believe their use is problematic (Diamond, Leckrone, Dennis, & Godley, 2006). Moreover, motivation for treatment and retention of those young persons referred by the legal system to substance abuse programs for marijuana disorders is lower than for those referred for other substances (Carroll, Sinha, & Easton, 2006). As MI specifically targets the core issue of ambivalence, its use with this population promotes the opportunity for the young person to at least have a voice in their treatment, despite their mandated status.

MI SPIRIT AND STRATEGIES

Using the Teen Marijuana Check-up (TMCU) as an illustration, we next discuss how MI can be used with young people who are smoking marijuana (Swan et al., 2008; Walker, Roffman, Stephens, Berghuis, & Kim, 2006). Intended to reach adolescents who do not identify themselves as in need of treatment, the TMCU includes recruitment strategies tailored to reach the concerned adolescent marijuana smoker (although many of our participants were not concerned about their use but were interested in asking questions about marijuana) and a two-session MET (motivational enhancement therapy) intervention delivered in high schools.

Recruitment Strategies

To encourage voluntary participation, several barriers to participation can be reduced with the incorporation of MI-informed principles. First, advertisements should not label the intervention as "treatment," nor should they refer to those interested as having "a problem" with marijuana. Rather, all young persons with "questions or concerns about marijuana" can be invited to participate. Unbalanced or overly negative information about marijuana needs to be avoided, confidentiality protected, and parental consent ideally not required (see Walker et al., 2006).

Advertisement

Advertisement of your program, such as in the TMCU, can occur mainly through classroom or community presentations during the school day to help reach the adolescent group. Use of interactive and balanced presentations providing information on myths and facts of marijuana use can be delivered first, followed by encouraging youth to participate and discuss what they've "heard about" marijuana. Use of your OARS skills to elicit these contributions is helpful at this initial stage of engagement. For example, eliciting questions such as "What are your thoughts about marijuana?" and all answers, even those that may sound seemingly naive, such as "It's cool—there's nothing else we can do," are respected. All and any youth participation should be reinforced with use of reflective listening skills (i.e., "Using pot isn't really a worry for you right now").

Next, the nature and purpose of your program should be discussed. In the TMCU we next ask each teen to complete a confidential form evaluating the informational program. Students who are interested in being contacted by one of our staff to hear more about the program are instructed to write their name on the evaluation form. As all forms are collected, this acts as a confidential way for young people to indicate their interest in the program. Confidentiality is further protected through careful and thoughtful protocols for contacting students. For example, youth may be called out of class by project staff using passes signed by school staff (i.e., those not associated with the TMCU project), or they may be asked to meet at a later time when caregivers are not present. Thus, interest and participation in your intervention, as in the TMCU, remains confidential. As in all of your work with young persons (see Chapter 21 on ethics), careful, respectful, and autonomy-supporting attitudes should be at the forefront of your interactions with teens before and during sessions. For example, a commonly conveyed message during interactions includes the following: "We're here to talk, but what you decide to do with your marijuana use is completely up to you."

Assessment Strategies

After consenting to participate, teens can be assessed using a computerized questionnaire. The assessment includes quantity and frequency of use, marijuana abuse and dependence symptoms, treatment history for substance use or mental health, perceived costs and benefits from reducing marijuana use, self-efficacy for avoiding marijuana use, and important goals. Questions you may consider include: How many days have you used marijuana in the past 60 days? How often do you use marijuana on the days you use? Have you ever received treatment or counseling for your use of marijuana? What might be the costs to you of reducing your marijuana use? What might be the benefits to you of reducing your use?

Feedback Strategies

After engaging the young person, employing the principles and techniques of MI may include the provision of personalized feedback. One tool we have developed and found helpful in the TCMU includes the Personal Feedback Report. The Personal Feedback Report, comprised of information from the assessment, includes descriptive information regarding the participant's use, normative data on marijuana, money spent on marijuana, consequences of use, social supports, benefits of reducing use, and future goals. Youth are often surprised by the normative information provided on what percentage of youth their age have used marijuana. Questions can include the following: "What do you make of this?" "What does it mean to be using more than most teens your age?" With regard to future goals, the youth can be asked: "How does your marijuana use fit in with your goal of going to college?" "What else could you do with the money you spend on marijuana?" "How might you benefit if you chose to reduce your use?"

Normative Feedback

Young persons are often more strongly influenced by their peers than by adults. Research on perceived social norms in general suggests that (1) one's beliefs about peers' risky behaviors are related to personal behavior (Borsari & Carey, 2001); (2) people tend to overestimate risk behaviors, especially those who are engaging in risky behavior (Baer, Stacy, & Larimer, 1991); and (3) personalized feedback containing accurate prevalence information is an effective intervention for changing normative misperceptions and behavior (Lewis & Neighbors, 2006). Normative misperceptions do occur with marijuana use, and overestimating marijuana use by friends and peers is related to personal use and problems associated with substance use among college students (Kilmer et al., 2006).

The provision of normative feedback on marijuana use can illuminate to the young person how their behavior is "outside the norm." Although norms data is often received with disbelief, rolling with resistance is an effective strategy to disseminate this information and help to maintain interest in the conversation with the practitioner. In addition, presenting norms data along with a short explanation of the origin of the data can offset the skepticism often reported by young persons. For example, if the data are coming from a large longitudinal data set, an explanation of the ways the researchers promoted honest responses from participants can help to ease explanations, and reduce comments such as "Those kids obviously lied." Other common responses to norms data include "That can't be right" or "Everyone I hang out with smokes pot." When these responses occur, practitioners can still respond in an affirmative and a nonconfrontive manner, while avoiding heavy defense of the data or argument with the young person. For example, useful statements can include: "That makes a lot of sense. We tend to hang out with people who are interested in the same kinds of things. So you *may not* be hanging out with the people who don't use." Or "So these numbers don't fit your experience."

Use an Empathic and Eliciting Style

Young people rarely have opportunities to talk with an adult about drug use in a noncombative or nondidactic manner, and an empathic and eliciting style centered on personal perspectives of use serves to build rapport and trust. For young persons displaying minimal communication, (i.e., the nontalkers), the elicitation of experiences and thoughts about drug use through open questions can truly enhance your interactions and their engagement in treatment. Once a young person understands that his or her perspective is being sought for the sole reason that it is valued, the likelihood of that person becoming more comfortable with talking can be substantially increased.

Incorporate Affirmations

Young people infrequently talk with adults about their drug use, and affirmations serve not only to establish rapport but also to convey the message that they are worthwhile individuals. For example, many adolescents have expressed to us their concerns about being pigeonholed as a "pothead" or "stoner." Noticing and acknowledging the young person as more than a "marijuana user" by offering praise for intrinsic strengths (i.e.,"You're thoughtful about your future," or "Being a good friend is important to you") can promote an honest evaluation of personal use habits. Similarly, your incorporation of affirmations conveys the spirit of MI: being non-judgmental and promoting self-efficacy to reduce and sustain from use. For example, change can appear more possible when the strengths of the individual are emphasized and explored (i.e., "I can see you work hard at something when you've set your mind to it. I bet if you decide to make a change with your use, you'll do it."

Decisional Balance Strategies

Low motivation to change is common among adolescents with marijuana use disorders. The decisional balance exercise can be helpful in exploring ambivalence around use. The pros and cons exercise allows for the respectful and goal-directed asking of how marijuana use "works" for the young person. By providing a platform for voicing the benefits of use, a discussion can be forged to explore potential downsides. For example, when costs of use are explored after the pros, the "Yeah, but . . ." statements can be minimized when the practitioner actively uses reflective listening skills. The decisional balance can further pave the way for examining the aspects of use with which the teen is dissatisfied, as well as the consequences of continued use.

Develop Discrepancy

Developing discrepancy in any substance misuse habit is a skill well worth acquiring in working with young populations. At first glance, many young persons do not perceive their marijuana use as problematic. With gentle yet tailored discussions about use, discrepancy can be explored between actual use and current values or future aspirations. Common topic areas for developing discrepancy include money spent on marijuana, social support, and future goals.

For example, money spent on marijuana can be calculated based on the teen's report (e.g., $75 a month on marijuana equates to $900 annually). So after eliciting reactions about cost, you might ask: "What else could you see yourself doing with 900 dollars?" Considering other meaningful items money could be put toward can create dissonance about spending money on marijuana or reveal ways in which drug use is interfering with financial goals.

Asking a young person to think about social supports and to identify the four most important people in their lives is also a fruitful exercise for developing discrepancy. Guiding a discussion to explore how those important people view the young person's use and what they would think if they continued or cut down can be enlightening. Common questions to ask include: "Which of these people know that you use marijuana?" "How come you haven't told some of them?" "What might they be concerned about if they knew you were using?" These questions can stimulate thinking about the young person's values. For example, a young person may be very open about his or her use with friends, but not with an admired adult. Gently probing for reasons as to why the behavior is kept secret from certain persons in the young person's inner support circle can magnify these discrepancies. The following is a brief example of probing with an MI style.

YOUNG PERSON: My coach wouldn't approve of me smoking.

PRACTITIONER: She would make a different choice for you. Why?

YOUNG PERSON: Well, I guess she'd be freaked out that it's going to affect how I play and probably thinks it's not healthy.

PRACTITIONER: She's concerned about your health and your performance. What do you think about that?

YOUNG PERSON: I know it doesn't help. After a weekend of smoking, I feel really slow on the field and I cough more.

PRACTITIONER: It sounds like your coach really cares about you and wants what is best for your future. Soccer is important to you and you know smoking isn't helping your performance any.

Looking toward Future Goals

Looking toward future goals can also be helpful in developing discrepancy and building motivation to change. First, you ask the young person to name five important current and future goals. Second, you consider each goal in relation to the teen's current use. Finally, the young person is asked how continuing or quitting use might affect each goal. For example, if the youth's goal is to attend college, you might ask questions about the effects of continued use (i.e., "If your use remained the same, how might it affect your goal of going to college?"), as well as reducing or terminating use (i.e., "How might reducing or quitting affect this goal?").

RESEARCH IMPLICATIONS

For young persons with marijuana use disorders, MET has been evaluated as a stand-alone intervention and as one component of a multicomponent intervention including CBT. The Cannabis Youth Treatment study was the largest controlled trial of therapies for adolescents (Dennis et al., 2004). Five sessions of MET/CBT were shown to have similar efficacy for reducing marijuana use as more intensive treatments, such as the community reinforcement approach, multidimensional family therapy, and MET/CBT with family support network. Five sessions of MET/CBT were also demonstrated to be more cost-effective than longer interventions.

MET has also been adapted as a brief intervention for young persons not seeking treatment. McCambridge and Strang (2004) recruited 200 students ages 16 to 20 who used marijuana or stimulants weekly in a U.K. population. Students randomized to receive one session of MI reduced their use of marijuana, alcohol, and cigarettes more than students in the assessment-only control condition. The MI intervention did not involve personalized feedback but instead consisted of the counselor using MI skills. A menu of topics guided the session selected by the counselor to meet the individual needs of each student. Topics included areas of conversation related to building motivation to change such as pros and cons of use, consequences of use and how they relate to values and goals, and a decisional balance exercise. Our own work with the Teen Marijuana Check-Up and the work of others demonstrated the success of a one- to two-session MET intervention to elicit voluntary participation and marijuana reductions from non-treatment-seeking teens (Berghuis, Swift, Roffman, Stephens, & Copeland, 2006; Martin & Copeland, 2008; Walker et al., 2006). These interventions included the provision of personalized feedback and the counselor's use of MI skills.

The findings of controlled trials of MI interventions delivered to young persons who are abusing marijuana are promising. However, further randomized controlled trials, particularly in non-treatment settings, are needed. Future studies will be needed to examine the most optimal formats (e.g., in-person, computerized, web-based, via telephone, or some combination) for delivering brief MI interventions to adolescent marijuana users. More also needs to be known about how to effectively respond to clients who are at an early phase of motivation to change (e.g., in-school counseling and/or support groups, computerized or web-based interventions, or some combination of these).

CHAPTER 11

❋ ❋ ❋ ❋

The Juvenile Justice System

L. A. R. Stein

SCOPE OF THE PROBLEM

About 153,384 adolescents are incarcerated per year (Puzzanchera, 2003) in the United States. Young people in the justice system have multiple mental health difficulties, including substance use. High rates of substance use disorders have been documented among detainees, especially those involving alcohol and marijuana (McClelland, Elkington, Teplin, & Abram, 2004). Similarly, high rates of psychiatric disorders have been found among these adolescents (Teplin, Abram, McClelland, Dulan, & Mericle, 2002), including affective, anxiety, and conduct disorders (Teplin, 2001). In addition, these adolescents engage in a variety of behaviors putting themselves and others at risk for serious deleterious outcomes.

Adolescents in the justice system appear to be at high risk for driving under or being a passenger with someone under the influence of substances (DUI and PUI) (Stein et al., 2006). One study of incarcerated adolescents (N = 130) indicated that 58% and 81%, respectively, had engaged in DUI and PUI related to alcohol or marijuana during the last 12 months (Stein, 2004). Another study found that 95% of adolescent detainees engaged in unprotected vaginal or anal sex (Teplin, Mericle, McClelland, & Abram, 2003). Incarcerated adolescents appear to use condoms inconsistently (Nagamune & Bellis, 2002; Rickman, Lodico, & DiClemente, 1994), are more likely to exchange sex for drugs (Wood & Shoroye, 1993), and have sex while under the influence of substances (Otto-Salaj, Gore-Felton, McGarvey, & Canterbury II, 2002) than nonincarcerated adolescents.

Although there is a need for treatment targeting substance use and related risky behaviors, adolescents in the justice system may be poorly engaged in available services (Melnick, De Leon, Hawke, Jainchill, & Kressel, 1997; Nissen, 2006; Prochaska et al., 1994). In addition, such services are often unavailable (Nissen, 2006; Thornberry, Tolnay, Flanagan, & Glynn, 1991; Young, Dembo, & Henderson, 2007). Similarly, services for families of justice system–involved adolescents are often unavailable (Young et al., 2007), and when they are, these families may exhibit a lack of treatment investment (Perkins-Dock, 2001). Adding to these difficulties in availability and engagement is the fast-paced nature of justice settings: Many adolescents are detained for only a matter of days, and similarly, incarcerated adolescents are sometimes released unexpectedly.

WHY MI?

MI is brief, meets adolescents where they are in terms of interest in change, is developmentally consistent with adolescent strivings for autonomy, and addresses mechanisms thought to be important to change (e.g., self-efficacy).

Because it is brief, MI is well suited for settings with few resources. MI is also indicated for people high in anger or hostility, which are common emotions in the criminal justice system (Karno & Longabaugh, 2004; Waldron, Slesnick, Brody, Turner, & Peterson, 2001). For example, as many as 40% of juveniles show significant anger when initially detained (Stein, Slavet, Gingras, & Golembeske, 2004). Additional evidence supporting use of MI for adolescents is provided elsewhere in this text.

MI SPIRIT AND STRATEGIES

Consideration of the ecology of the justice systems in which these adolescents are found is critical. For example, staff members may find it uneasy to both answer to the court and act to serve in an adolescent's best interests while utilizing MI. Many factors come into consideration at this juncture, including the philosophy of the staff member (authoritarian vs. collaborative), professional affiliation (agent of the court vs. social welfare), background and training (criminal justice vs. social work), work climate (punitive vs. rehabilitative orientation), and quality of supervision, to name a few of the more salient factors. The careful use of MI by legal and correctional practitioners may maximize therapeutic effects of the law and minimize antitherapeutic consequences of the law (called therapeutic jurisprudence; see Birgden, 2004; Feldstein & Ginsberg, 2006).

Probation/parole officers (POs) are a group working within justice system settings who might effectively deliver MI. POs attempt to engage offenders in discussions about offending, and address those areas that may put the adolescent in danger of re-offending. The difficulty may lie in the PO determining what content to report (or not) to the court. The adolescent's good-faith efforts to engage in a process with the PO to comply with the court and take steps toward beginning a more prosocial life can allow POs to use discretion in reporting infractions (K. McKenna, Assistant Director, RI Juvenile Probation, personal communication, October 15, 2007). When used well by POs, MI allows adolescents to challenge themselves by examining their own behavior (Mann, Ginsberg, & Weeks, 2002), as well as hear in their own words the possibility of a different life and the reasons to seek one. Of utmost importance is informing and reminding the adolescent of the parameters of confidentiality, the nature and purpose of the discussions, and the PO's role within the local ecology. Persons interested in the ethics associated with use of MI in such situations should consult Miller and Rollnick (2002) as well as Part III of this text.

The spirit of MI, with its focus on empathy, its nonjudgmental stance, and its emphasis on personal choice, contrasts well with environments that may be perceived as punitive and confrontational. While MI strategies in general are relevant for this population to promote engagement in treatment, youth seem to respond particularly well to certain strategies utilized during MI.

Double-Sided Reflection with Decisional Balance

Adolescents involved in the justice system often respond well to the double-sided reflection and summary provided at the close of the decisional balance exercises. It appears powerful for them to hear in their own words why they engage in certain behaviors, such as substance use and sexual risk, and yet they can clearly identify significant difficulties associated with their behaviors. For example: "So it sounds like smoking marijuana is a way for you to relax and socialize with friends, yet on the other hand you said it's upset your mother. Now that you think about it, most of your car accidents happened after you smoked. I can see you're struggling with this situation—it's not easy when you consider the good and not-so-good things that come out of using marijuana." As evidenced by this example, when an adolescent's struggle is acknowledged, it assists in not only conveying empathy, but also in guiding the conversation to the central target areas of motivation and change.

Rolling with Resistance

As noted in previous chapters, personalized feedback is a common tool used to address the substance use problems found in this population. Rolling with resistance during the personalized feedback is of utmost importance, for frequently these adolescents are incredulous during normative feedback. Within a context mandated to maintain custody and control, adolescents seem to look forward to the MI because it is one of the few instances in which they clearly experience empathy and respect for their autonomy. During the feedback session, an adolescent might comment, "I know you want me to stop, but I won't—they can lock me up but nobody can make me stop once I'm out of here." Responding to this with, "I hear you, only you can make decisions for you," can be quite effective to help facilitate their continued engagement and reduce the potential of counter-motivational behaviors.

Supporting Self-Efficacy

Being astute at recognizing and addressing premature self-efficacy is important. Occasionally, adolescents will feel overconfident in their ability to reduce or stop engaging in their risk-taking behaviors, should they choose to do so. Probing for previous attempts at reducing such behaviors and what made it difficult is helpful. Alternatively, it is also helpful to assist adolescents in re-creating a very detailed scenario in which they may have engaged in risky behaviors before, and then review what might be difficult about altering their decisions and actions in the future. These discussions can be followed by use of creative questions to help build and support self-efficacy:

> "What might you imagine doing differently?"
> "What would it take to get you there? May I make some suggestions? . . ."
> "It sounds like you've really thought about this now and have some good options. What about you makes you think you can do this?"
> "Tell me about something you've been able to accomplish in your past."

Integrating the Use of Rewards

After meeting goals, it is recommended that adolescents reward themselves. It is important to convey the idea that rewards are special and not a regular occurrence, as well as that they should be somewhat meaningful to the adolescent and relatively under his or her control to administer. Within this setting, it is sometimes tricky to identify such a reward. In addition, rewarding one's self in this fashion can often be foreign to these adolescents; they frequently express surprise at or disbelief in such a principle. Once explained, however, they seem to be able to identify any number of rewards, including extra dessert, writing a letter home, drawing a picture, rereading a letter from home, asking a parent to bring in fast-food or music (with facility approval), or even pausing to take pride in the accomplishment itself.

Addressing Peers

Discussions tailored to help the adolescent identify and understand the mutual impact peers have on each other can be effective; yet frequently adolescents have difficulty seeing the impact that another's risk-taking behaviors have on them. While adolescents may express a desire to change risky behaviors, to do so they are often faced with the difficult choice of having to reduce contact with risk-taking friends. One effective strategy for helping the adolescent to understand the mutual impact of peers involves the use of normative feedback. For example, in the case of an adolescent using methamphetamines: "You think 9/10 adolescents your age use, but really it's only about 2/10. You might think it's that high because *you* hang out with friends who use, but it's important to know that most people your age don't use." Listening carefully to adolescents and providing reflections that might assist them in reevaluating peer groups is also helpful: "I hear you, marijuana is a way to have fun with others and you wonder who you will be able to hang out with if you're not using. I'm wondering what you think your friend, James, does? He doesn't use anymore." Alternatively: "You sound pretty angry your friends have dropped you since you've been inside—you've even questioned whether they care about you, and just use you for drugs. I'm wondering how you might find friends with other interests aside from drugs, and other ways to use your time. I know you want to learn a trade to support your child—how might that lead to meeting new people who don't have time for drugs?"

RESEARCH IMPLICATIONS

MI has been used with adult offenders (for a brief review, see Feldstein & Ginsburg, 2006), but well-controlled studies are relatively rare. Although studies have only just begun to examine using MI to enhance motivation (e.g., to reduce substance use in justice system–involved persons), the results are encouraging (Davis, Baer, Saxon, & Kivlahan, 2003; Ginsburg, 2000; Harper & Hardy, 2000; Stein & Lebeau-Craven, 2002; Woodall, Delaney, Kunitz, Westerberg, & Zhao, 2007). In addition, although one review indicated modest or no effects for MI on adult offenders, methodological factors may well explain such findings (Ginsburg, Mann, Rotgers, & Weekes, 2002).

Several studies on adolescents have recruited large proportions of justice system–involved participants (about 33–60%), with promising results for the use of MI (see Breslin, Li, Sdao-Jarvie, Tupker, & Ittig-Deland, 2002; Dennis et al., 2004). Well-controlled studies with specific focus on incarcerated adolescents are emerging, with results favoring the efficacy of MI. In one randomized study ($N = 130$), as compared to relaxation training

(RT), MI was found to significantly reduce negative attitudes and behavior in adolescents subsequently enrolled in facility standard care (Stein et al., 2006b).

In a related study (N = 105; Stein et al., 2006a), as compared to RT, adolescents who received MI had lower rates of drinking and driving, and of being a passenger in a car with someone who had been drinking, but effects were moderated by levels of depression. At low levels of depression, MI evidenced lower rates of these behaviors; at high levels of depression, effects for MI and RT were equivalent. Similar patterns were found for marijuana-related risky driving, but effects were nonsignificant. These investigators also found (N = 114) that at lower levels of depressive symptoms, as compared to RT, adolescents randomly assigned to MI reported significantly fewer episodes of unprotected sex in general and unprotected sex while using marijuana (Rosengard et al., 2007).

Finally, this group conducted a pilot study of MI delivered to incarcerated adolescents and their families (Slavet et al., 2005). Results suggest that this MI-based treatment positively impacted families (effect sizes were generally in the medium range). After the intervention, adolescents were more confident in their ability to resist drug use and parents were more confident in their ability to impact their adolescents' risky behaviors. Parents and adolescents both reported being highly satisfied with this intervention. A more recent study with adolescent detainees (Schmiege, Broaddus, Levin, & Bryan, 2009) compared (1) group-based MI for alcohol use and group-based psychosocial treatment targeting risky sex (GMI + GPI), (2) GPI alone, and (3) group-based information only (INFO) and found that GMI+GPI was superior over INFO in reducing risky sexual behavior at a 3-month follow-up (N = 315).

Although these studies on incarcerated and detained juveniles and their families offer significant support for MI, it is important that such results be replicated in other settings. Work on moderators and mediators (mechanisms of action) is needed to understand how MI may effect change for this population, as well as to make tailored and more efficient versions of MI in this setting. Given the crucial need to engage disenfranchised families in environments with limited resources, further large-scale investigation of family-based MI is warranted. Also, work is needed on use of MI during *transition to* and *maintenance in* communities. Future publications will address impact on alcohol/marijuana use reductions (as presented by Stein, 2004). Finally, investigators may wish to study the delivery of MI by staff members employed within justice system settings, and how best to transmit MI to maintain its impact on adolescents and their families. This study may be especially critical because current dissemination of recommendations indicates the use of taped sessions to be reviewed under supervision (see Martino et al., 2006). However, use of such recordings may be discouraged or disallowed in justice settings.

CHAPTER 12

＊ ＊ ＊ ＊

Sexual Risk Reduction

Juline Koken, Angulique Outlaw, and Monique Green-Jones

SCOPE OF THE PROBLEM

Adolescence and emerging adulthood has been identified as a period when many experiment with risky behaviors, including sexual behavior. According to the 2007 Youth Risk Behavior Surveillance Survey (YRBSS), 47.8% of high school students have had sexual intercourse, and 7.1% reported first sexual intercourse before age 13 (Centers for Disease Control and Prevention [CDC], 2008b). Although education and the provision of information regarding the potential consequences of sexual risk-taking behavior appears a logical method of intervention, changing the risky practices of young persons is much more complex (Greene, Krcmar, Walters, Rubin, & Hale, 2000).

According to the 2007 YRBSS, 39% of currently sexually active high school students did not use a condom during last sexual intercourse and only 16% reported using the pill as a form of contraception (CDC, 2008b). Subsequently, these risky contraception practices have increased the prevalence of sexually transmitted infections (STIs) in young persons. Chlamydia rates for persons 15 to 19 and 20 to 24 years of age continue to increase, as have gonorrhea rates for the third consecutive year (CDC, 2007). The high prevalence of these STIs indicates a dangerous pattern of sexual risk behavior that increases the vulnerability of this population to acquiring and transmitting HIV. Indeed, an estimated 13% of those receiving a diagnosis of HIV/AIDS in 2004 were youth between the ages of 13 and 24

(CDC, 2008a). Emerging adults (ages 18–25) (Arnett, 2000, 2001) have the highest rates of risk behaviors and STIs compared to other developmental periods, and thus the lack of adequate and impactful intervention remains problematic.

Sexual Risk among Marginalized Populations

The highest rates of sexual activity occur among minority youth (i.e., African American young adults) (Park et al., 2006); and these populations disproportionately represent the majority of HIV cases, as well as the highest STI rates in the country. In addition to these sexual risks, it is well documented that minority status in the United States correlates with other fundamental determinants of health status such as poverty, lack of access to quality health care, reduced health-care-seeking behavior, illicit drug use, and living in communities with high prevalence of STIs and HIV (CDC, 2007). The disparity in rates of HIV and STIs between white and ethnic minority young persons is alarming and indicates an urgent need to prioritize the development of effective interventions for these groups.

According to a recent survey (Weiss Weiwel, 2009), the young men who have sex with men (YMSM) of color constitute the largest group of newly diagnosed HIV infections. The CDC found that the rates of new infections among black males in 2006 were more than *seven times* the rate of new infections among white males. An analysis of annual mean rates of HIV incidence among men who have sex with men (MSM) (Stall et al., 2009) found that if the current mean rate of new infection is sustained, HIV prevalence among MSM in North America will reach 40% by the time these men reach age 40. These statistics indicate an urgent need for effective, tailored, culturally responsive interventions targeting sexual risk behavior among YMSM and MSM of color.

The empirical literature has substantiated various developmental and adjustment problems experienced by emerging adult lesbian, gay, bisexual, transgender, and questioning (LGBTQ) persons, including risk of suicide, harassment or even violence at school (Safe Schools Coalition of Washington, 1999), behavioral issues, and substance use and abuse (Anhalt & Morris, 1998). Negative consequences stemming from life challenges (e.g., coming out to family members and friends, victimization due to sexual orientation) can pose an additional stressor for these youth and increases their vulnerability to risk behaviors (Anhalt & Morris, 1998; Rosario, Hunter, Maguen, Gwadz, & Smith, 2001). For example, one study found that sexual risk behavior was associated with depression in YMSM (Perdue, Hagan, Thiede, & Valleroy, 2003). Thus, there is a need for culturally tailored risk reduction interventions to decrease risk behaviors among marginalized youth.

WHY MI?

MI is an ideal method for working with youth engaging in sexual risk behaviors who may be more focused on the potential benefits of such behaviors than the potential consequences (Parsons, Siegel, & Cousins, 1997) or who may feel they are less likely than others to be exposed to HIV (Chapin, 2000). MI complements the sexual developmental issues unique to young people. For example, this period is a crucial time when young persons may be developing their sexual identity, experimenting sexually, and potentially experimenting with substance use during sexual activity. During this time youth are establishing their independence, and sexual behavior may be an expression of their maturing self. MI, with its emphasis on reinforcing autonomy and collaboration, can significantly reduce defensiveness and psychological reactance commonly seen when adolescents and young adults feel pressured to change. Thus, MI may enhance the likelihood that the young person will participate in a sexual risk reduction intervention.

MI SPIRIT AND STRATEGIES

The underlying "spirit" of MI (Miller & Rollnick, 2002) is especially helpful when working with young persons who engage in sexual risk behavior. Respecting the young person's right to self-determination (Autonomy) may help reduce resistance from clients who may already be defensive about discussing their sexuality and sexual behavior. Working with the young person on setting realistic goals (Collaboration) regarding safer sex, rather than imposing your own agenda may further strengthen your alliance with the young person. Finally, you empower the young person by looking to his or her expertise and experience as a resource for ideas about how to reduce sexual risk behavior (Evocation), rather than viewing the client's past behavior as "bad."

The spirit of MI is particularly powerful when working with marginalized youth of color, sexual minority youth, and young persons who have experienced the loss of basic freedoms, such as those who have been placed in detention facilities. While the importance of emphasizing the right to make choices about one's own body and sexual behaviors is essential, you may need to work at maintaining an even, nonjudgmental stance even when young people discuss their sexual behavior in explicit or confrontational ways. The emphasis on the youth's autonomy may be helpful when working with youth exhibiting these behaviors.

The "spirit" of MI may also act as a protective factor for preventing or alleviating practitioner burnout when working with youth at high risk of contracting HIV. You may feel a sense of personal responsibility and protectiveness toward young clients, and this may sometimes interfere with the focus on the client's perception of their sexual behavior, autonomy, and inner resources for change. When practicing the "spirit of MI" in work with young people, you shift the focus back to the client. Thus, remaining cognizant of the young person's autonomy, and recognizing the strengths and resources they possess, may result in greater job satisfaction and lower risk of burnout (Osborn, 2004).

Agenda Setting and Menu of Options

Many risk behaviors are concurrent (e.g., engaging in unprotected sex while under the influence of substances, multiple partners), and several studies have effectively used MI to address these multiple issues. However, it may be challenging to focus on multiple behaviors within a brief counseling program. One way you may manage this is by targeting the interplay and impact of such risk behaviors on the young person's personal goals and values. You must have a clear plan for discussing target behaviors with young persons even when they may be resistant to doing so. Balancing these client-centered and directive skills is one of the challenges of practicing MI, and use of the agenda-setting strategy can facilitate this balance.

Sexual risk behaviors can include many facets such as unprotected sex, sex under the influence of substances, bartering sex for drugs or money, or having multiple partners. Limiting target behaviors to one or two can also serve to make the session more directed and more goal-focused. Consider the agenda-setting technique described in Chapter 3. You might try incorporating an agenda into a session's "opening statement," such as this: "I'm glad to see you today. I was hoping that in this session we could spend some time talking about your sexual life, your thoughts about what's risky or safe, and how things like alcohol or drug use may or may not be a part of sexual situations for you. I also want to let you know that I'm not here to judge your behavior or tell you what to do—ultimately, only *you* can decide what works best for you." You may also offer a menu of options from which the young person may choose ("today we can talk about your thoughts about your sexual behavior, your drug or alcohol use, or perhaps you have something you would like to discuss we haven't touched on yet. Where would you like to start?") and ask if there are additional issues he or she might like to address.

Decisional Balance

Eliciting change talk can sometimes be challenging, particularly when addressing sexual behavior issues with young people who are not ready to change. Two MI strategies helpful in handling potential resistance with such clients are the "decisional balance" and "siding with the negative."

A decisional balance is a classic strategy for exploring the positive and negative aspects of a behavior by explicitly placing the client in a position of expertise and authority. Most young persons find this activity easy to grasp and surprisingly powerful. You can use a piece of paper and ask the young person to list the "pros" and "cons" of the target behavior, or this can be done verbally. For example, you might ask, "what are some of the things you enjoy about having sex without a condom?" Starting with the positive and including the negative aspects of their behavior during the decisional balance can also successfully help the young person better focus on their perceptions about the benefits *and* consequences of their risk behaviors. Furthermore, this strategy also often leads to an increase in change talk and avoids inciting resistance, as a result of the emphasis placed on the young person, and not your views about the behavior.

Siding with the Negative

The "siding with the negative" strategy is useful for young people who may not view their sexual risk behavior as a problem or who are explicitly resistant to change. Based on the assumption that "all arguments have two sides," this strategy involves avoiding being the person arguing in favor of change, especially with young people who may be accustomed to being told what to do by various authority figures in their lives. The goal is to present the reasons why the young person may be reluctant to change as well as to emphasize her or his personal right to choose not to change and to experience the potential consequences of their decisions. For example, if you voice an opinion for one side of an argument (i.e., the difficulties involved in consistent condom use), the young person is more likely to take up an opposing position (i.e., discuss reasons why consistent condom use can be accomplished). By voicing their reasons for being reluctant to change, the young person may naturally take in the reasons why change could be positive.

Accepting the Young Person's Autonomy: Letting Go of Expertise

Two common challenges in practicing MI with young persons engaging in high-risk behaviors involves letting go of the expert/educator model of practice and fully accepting the principles of MI spirit, particularly autonomy. When you feel a great deal of concern about the young person's sexual risk behaviors, it may be tempting to revert to an educational and advice-heavy style of practice. Such an approach can elicit resistant behaviors, as well as place you at risk for work-related burnout and disengagement from the young people you are seeking to help.

RESEARCH IMPLICATIONS

Research on MI as an intervention for sexual risk behavior has shown promise, although to date, few published studies have focused specifically on marginalized youth. MI appears to be most effective for sexual risk behavior by increasing self-efficacy for condom use and safer sex negotiation between casual sex partners (Semple, Patterson, & Grant, 2004), targeting concurrent substance use (Shoptaw, Reback, Froshch, & Rawson, 1998), and when delivered to individuals in the earliest stages of change in brief doses (Picciano, Roffman, Kalichman, Rutledge, & Berghuis, 2001). LaBrie, Pederson, Thompson, and Earleywine (2008) found that a brief decisional balance intervention (a component of MI) was effective in promoting condom use among a sample of heterosexual college males. Ingersoll and colleagues (2005) found that a brief single MI session was effective in reducing alcohol consumption and increasing contraception use among college-aged women. Finally, Naar-King and colleagues (2008) examined the maintained effects of MET on risk behaviors and viral load for youth living with HIV (YLH). Results suggested that reductions in viral load and alcohol use were maintained after the termination of treatment; there were no improvements in condom use. Although there have been no published studies on MI for sexual risk reduction, a study using MI to encourage HIV counseling and testing in African American YMSM was recently completed and results are promising (Outlaw, Naar-King, Parsons, Green-Jones, & Secord, 2010).

MI-based interventions for sexual risk reduction with youth require more investigation. Research with larger samples of minority youth, specifically minority YMSM, is needed to determine the efficacy of motivational interventions in reducing sexual risk behaviors. MI may also be useful when determining youth motivation for participation in intensive, multisession interventions (e.g., diffusion of effective behavioral interventions, or DEBIs). MI may be useful as a preparatory intervention for more intensive interventions. MI in combination with cognitive-behavioral therapy and skills training has shown promise in reducing substance use (Parsons, Rosof, Punzalan, & Di Maria, 2005). Finally, more components of risk reduction strategies need to be incorporated into future research, especially for YLH. As the incidence of HIV infection continues to rise, particularly among minority youth and minority YMSM, the need for effective intervention strategies is urgent. MI is an empirically validated brief intervention that may be especially appropriate for working with marginalized youth. MI may blend well with multisession, intensive interventions, and shows promise for future research and programming.

CHAPTER 13

✳ ✳ ✳ ✳

Smoking

Kimberly Horn

SCOPE OF THE PROBLEM

After steadily decreasing in the last decade, teen smoking rates have stabilized at levels significantly above previously established national targets. The most recent YRBSS reveals that many states are beginning to observe a leveling off of progress in youth smoking trends (Agency for Healthcare Research and Quality [AHRQ], 2008). Current cigarette use among high school youth remained unchanged from 2003 to 2007 following an increase from 27.5% in 1991 to 36.4% in 1997, and subsequently a significant decline to 21.9% in 2003 (AHRQ, 2008). Consistently, teen smoking cessation remains a U.S. public health priority (Centers for Disease Control and Prevention [CDC], 2006; Eaton et al., 2008). Adolescence is the critical life period for smoking initiation; 70% of adult smokers smoked daily by age 18 (CDC, 2006). Youth who smoke may experience increased respiratory distress and illness and decreased physical fitness (Ramsey et al., 2008). Alcohol and illicit drug use, violence, stress, depression, high-risk sexual behaviors, and cognitive deficits also are associated with adolescent smoking (Ramsey et al., 2008; Sussman, 2005; Wang et al., 1998). Most youth who smoke continue smoking into adulthood, thereby elevating their lifetime risk for cardiovascular disease (Prokhorov et al., 2006; Ramsey et al., 2008) and several types of cancer, especially lung cancer (Jemal, Chu, & Tarone, 2001).

A common response to youth smoking is to convince young people to avoid developing the habit rather than helping them to break the habit

(Backinger, Fagan, Matthews, & Grana, 2003; McDonald, Colwell, Backinger, Husten, & Maule, 2003; Milton, Maule, Backinger, & Gregory, 2003). Although prevention efforts are vital, they do not address the needs of adolescents and young adults who smoke and want to quit. Importantly, many habitual young smokers consider quitting. Research shows that a majority of high school smokers who ever smoked daily had tried quitting on their own (Backinger et al., 2003; Horn, Fernandes, Dino, Massey, & Kalsekar, 2003). Although most teen quit attempts are unsuccessful (Sussman, Sun, & Dent, 2006), research has uncovered a few available and effective cessation options to help teens achieve cessation (Grimshaw & Stanton, 2006; Sussman et al., 2006).

Research highlights the immediate need for effective and available cessation options for youth who want to quit smoking. Different from past versions, the most recent USDHHS Clinical Guidelines for Treating Tobacco Dependence (AHRQ, 2008) now provides recommendations for delivering effective teen cessation interventions. Critically, interventions for youth must be more than simple modifications of adult interventions. Effective youth intervention requires a focus on issues and topics highly relevant to teens, including use of teen-friendly language and concepts. Broadly, research suggests that teen smoking interventions should incorporate assertiveness and refusal skills training, discuss the manipulative tactics of tobacco advertising, involve parents and family members, and deal with family and peer pressure (Curry et al., 2007; Horn, Dino, Goldcamp, Kalsekar, & Mody, 2005).

The field demands a variety of intervention approaches for teens who smoke and want to quit. The most commonly used approaches are school-based group intervention programs (Horn et al., 2005; Sussman, Lichtman, Ritt, & Pallonen, 1999). Other approaches include clinic-based individual interventions, family-based programs, and Internet self-help programs (Grimshaw & Stanton, 2006; Sussman, 2002; Sussman et al., 1999). Although a sound research base exists in support of the efficacy of school-based programs such as Not On Tobacco (N-O-T; Horn et al., 2005) and Project EX (Sussman, Dent, & Lichtman, 2001), there is limited research on the feasibility and efficacy of other intervention approaches for youth. Thus, many questions about optimal approaches remain unanswered (Mermelstein, 2003). Although schools are critical venues for youth tobacco control, it is unrealistic to assume that school-based interventions can serve, and be suitable for, millions of U.S. teen smokers. Focusing only on schools and on intensive intervention limits access, particularly for high-risk teens who attend school infrequently, hold negative attitudes toward school, are dropouts, are detained, or attend schools with limited resources. Ideally, youth who smoke should be saturated with options for cessation in multiple settings—schools, churches, primary care settings, and other clinical and community settings.

WHY MI?

MI is a common method used to facilitate clinic-based brief smoking intervention (Miller & Rollnick, 2002), an emergent strategy for teen smokers (Brown et al., 2003; Colby et al., 1998). Brief intervention using MI facilitates (1) patient-centered negotiation where providers respond sensitively to patients' feelings about quitting smoking, especially motivational ambivalence; (2) consideration of patient values and preferences; and (3) shared decision making between the patient and provider (Miller & Sanchez, 1994; Werner, 1995). Some research indicates that motivational techniques may also hold promise for teen smoking cessation and reduction (Colby et al., 1998; Landowski, 1998), as they typically occur in a single "on-the-spot" intervention (usually less than 30 minutes). Many experts suggest that MI supports a population health approach to reach large numbers of teen smokers without the resource demands of multisession interventions. Moreover, and particularly important for teens, research suggests that MI may be acceptable to teens because of its brief duration and nonconfrontational and empathic approach (Landowski, 1998).

Some teens experience greater difficulty quitting than others. Compared to lighter smokers, for example, we know that teens who are heavier smokers are also more addicted, more likely to be embedded in social networks with other smokers, and have less confidence in and less motivation for quitting (Branstetter, Horn, Dino, & Jhang, 2009). MI provides "the hook" to address these types of issues. More specifically, MI can be (1) designed and implemented in developmentally appropriate ways, spanning a broad age range of youth, (2) tailored to individual and gender-specific needs, giving practitioners the flexibility with their target populations, and (3) combined with additional components (e.g., with educational materials and other specialized treatment programs). In addition, it is flexible and brief enough to use in a variety of settings and can reinforce efforts made in schools and communities. Such flexibility, for example, reduces some of the access barriers common to multisession school-based programs.

MI also addresses another problem encountered by multisession interventions with teens: high dropout rates. Critically, program dropout is associated with motivational ambivalence, which is a characteristic of heavily addicted smokers. MI can influence the uncertainty teens have about changing their smoking behaviors and may occur in a single, on-the-spot interaction. Teens are most likely to make smoking behavior changes when they perceive that it is a problem and when they feel they have the power to change. MI is particularly well suited for the difficult, resistant, and hard-to-reach youth because it is tailored to individual needs. Taken together, these factors suggest that MI may serve as a feasible method to promote smoking cessation or reduction among teens.

MI SPIRIT AND STRATEGIES

The tailored, supportive nature of MI is consistent with research indicating that social support is an important feature of effective smoking cessation intervention (Pust, Mohnen, & Schneider, 2008; Simons-Morton et al., 1999; Sussman, 2005). Goal setting, follow-up, and timing also are important aspects of MI (Graham & Fleming, 1998). Integral to using MI is an understanding of the transtheoretical model of change developed by Prochaska and DiClemente (Prochaska, DiClemente, & Norcross, 1992). According to this model, smokers can be classified into five stages of change: (1) precontemplation (no intention of quitting); (2) contemplation (thinking about quitting but have made no commitment); (3) preparation (planning to quit within 30 days and having made a serious quit attempt); (4) action (quit for 6 months or less); or (5) maintenance (quit for more than 6 months).

Illustrating how these principles are tailored for smoking intervention, Goldberg and colleagues (1994) found that a stage-based approach to smoking cessation promotes short-term movement through the stages. Research confirms that low motivation and low self-efficacy are related to low quit rates among teens (Branstetter et al., 2009). Stage movement, even if incremental, can move teens closer to complete cessation. More specifically, MI techniques are used to build motivational and decisional balance such that teen smokers' thoughts about and intentions for quitting are greater than before they encountered MI. Motivational approaches also offer flexibility of implementation and tailoring for a youth-centered approach across settings. For example, MI's portability permits use in schools, community centers, clinics, or other venues where youth frequent. Practitioners' busy schedules often prohibit them from implementing intensive multisession programs with teens—sometimes they choose to do nothing at all rather than provide a lengthy program. MI provides a compromise to this dilemma. It is also appropriate for a variety of subpopulations of smokers (e.g., males, females, LGBTQ, racial/ethnic, etc.). Although MI provides guidance for the essential elements, it is not so scripted that practitioners cannot incorporate their own knowledge and familiarity with the target group. Table 13.1 demonstrates possible applications and a guide for implementing MI as a teen smoking intervention.

RESEARCH IMPLICATIONS

Several studies demonstrate the potential impact of MI on teen smoking cessation and reduction in various settings, such as hospitals and emergency rooms, psychiatric facilities, as well as schools. A seminal study by Colby

TABLE 13.1. Motivational Interviewing for Teen Smokers

Principle	MI focus
Use an empathic style.	Use a warm, reflective, and understanding style throughout the interaction with a teen. Avoid aggressive, confrontational, or coercive methods. Be sensitive to current teen trends and pop language. It is essential that teens feel supported in their views and efforts, even if different than what you would choose for them. Sidestep resistance by being empathic rather than judgmental or confrontational about smoking. If the teen expresses anger or other emotions, reflect back the expressed emotion and take a less intense position. • "I understand that you felt angry when your parents grounded you for smoking. How do you think they should react to your smoking? What would you do if you were the parent?" • "I get that you don't want me to bug you about your smoking. What do you think is the best way to help someone think about quitting cigarettes?"
Develop discrepancy.	Following assessment of smoking status (e.g., smoking on ≥ 1 day in past 30 days = current smoker), it is important to help teens recognize and define their current smoking behaviors and how those behaviors may be inconsistent with other aspects of life they value. To bring attention to their current smoking behaviors, offer feedback on immediate risks or potential medical consequences associated with current smoking patterns. For example, relate smoking to problem indicators (e.g., carbon monoxide readings) and current health conditions or problems they may have (e.g., chronic respiratory infections). • "Have you noticed that you cough a lot in the mornings when you wake up?" • "Do you have difficulty tasting your food?" • "Compared to a year ago, do you seem to have more problems with your asthma? Are you more winded after you exercise?" Develop a discrepancy between the teen's values and his or her current behaviors related to smoking. For example, most teens value good health and may not attribute certain uncomfortable physical symptoms to smoking. As another more social-oriented example, most teens are interested in dating and may not consider that smoke-filled clothing may be a turn-off to other teens. • "What is important in your life right now? What value do you place on your health?" • "How do you think smoking might affect your dating life?"
Emphasize personal responsibility.	Place emphasis on the teen's responsibility and choice to quit or reduce smoking. • "What you do about your smoking is up to you—do you have a plan?"
Discuss pros and cons of change.	Assess the teen's willingness to make a quit attempt and his or her readiness to change. Lead teens to address the pros and cons of their habit. • "What are the downsides of smoking in your life?" • "What are the things you would miss about smoking?"

(cont.)

TABLE 13.1. *(cont.)*

Principle	MI focus
Ask permission to offer advice.	If willing to make a quit attempt, offer specific reasons why quitting is important based on information obtained during the interview or interaction. Reduction also may be discussed here. Have fact-based resources on hand. Teens will quickly notice if you lack knowledge.

- "Based on what you said earlier, quitting might help you in the following ways . . ."

Offer a variety of strategies for changing smoking behavior.

- "Here are some things you can try . . . [explain]"
  - Setting limits
  - Recognizing antecedents or physical prompts and cues
  - Learning coping skills and stress management

Use a visual cue card to aid discussions about various strategies and techniques (e.g., the Internet).

Offer self-help print or Internet materials to supplement advice and to help patients carry out strategies effectively.

Make referrals to intensive cessation programs or quit lines, social networking sites, or other Internet-based programs or resources.

Incorporate the use of current technologies whenever feasible (e.g., texting; text alerts; and applications from iPhones or other personal devices).

and colleagues (1998) found that MI for teen smoking cessation in a hospital setting significantly reduced smoking dependence and the number of days of reported smoking. Another study found that MI resulted in modest, but significant, short-term reductions in quantity and frequency of smoking relative to standard care among adolescent psychiatric patients (Brown et al., 2003). An emergency-room-based study by Horn, Dino, Hamilton, and Noerachmanto (2007) found a medium effect size for smoking reduction and a large effect size for percentage reduction. In 2009, a large-scale project, the Hutchinson Study of High School Smoking, proactively identified over 2,000 students in 50 high schools in Washington State. Students who received the telephone counseling intervention consisting of MI and cognitive-behavioral skills training achieved a more significant reduction in smoking at 7 days, 1 and 3 months since their last cigarette, as well as a greater prolonged abstinence over a 6-month period (Peterson et al., 2009). In summary, research suggests that MI may facilitate cessation and reduction. Critically, some of the most recent trials suggest that MI may have some value as a harm reduction approach and a bridge to complete cessation (Horn et al., 2007).

Few studies have examined the overall feasibility of clinic-based motivational behavior change strategies for teens (Brown et al., 2003; Horn, Dino, Hamilton, Noerachmanto, & Zhang, 2008), particularly in the settings for which they are most recommended (i.e., hospital clinics and emergency rooms). The lack of feasibility assessment has critical implications since interventions lacking implementation feasibility are unlikely to find widespread adoption, even if proven effective. Without a strong reference base for feasibility, practitioners who chose to use MI should take steps to assess and understand the potential feasibility of it in their target settings (Glasgow, Vogt, & Boles, 1999). Feasibility can be assessed by answering questions such as (Glasgow, Goldstein, Ockene, & Pronk, 2004; Mermelstein & Turner, 2006): "How much does it cost? What are the time requirements? Does it require staff training? Is there access to the target population? How much space is needed? Do we have the necessary equipment? Can we access program materials? Does the program require any additional services (e.g., transportation)?" Moreover, Glasgow and colleagues (1999) recommends that feasibility must address critical factors of teen reach, adolescent and practitioner acceptability, and ease of implementation. However, sometimes interventions may be effective under controlled conditions, but not feasible or acceptable in real-world clinical conditions. Other times, interventions may be mostly feasible and acceptable, but not effective in terms of complete cessation (Horn et al., 2008).

Following the recommendations of Glasgow and colleagues, a recent study (Horn et al., 2008) found MI to be feasible with teens in an emergency room setting—perhaps one of the most challenging settings to deliver interventions. The findings of Horn and colleagues (2008) underscore the importance of examining all facets of intervention programming. Crucial feasibility issues of reach, recruitment, and retention require in-depth investigation, especially in settings where practitioners attempt to reach high-risk or medically compromised youth.

Different settings may pose unique challenges. As noted by Horn and colleagues (2008), clinical settings such as emergency rooms may present distinct challenges concerning medical or psychiatric acuity. It may be necessary to administer motivational interventions among certain subgroups of teen patients with less severe symptoms or conditions. For example, many medical sites (e.g., emergency rooms or express clinics) across the United States now have mechanisms to "fast track" nonacute patients. Second, in contrast to school or community settings that expect long-term relationships with youth, other types of settings (e.g., medical settings) experience time-limited youth-provider relationships. Motivational interventions may require a tailored approach to establish trust and to retain participants for follow-up contact because there are no established relationships in place (Wolfenden, Campbell, Walsh, Raoul, & Wiggers, 2003). Prior to implementation, researchers and practitioners should carefully and strategically plan to address reach and recruitment barriers that may be unique or characteristic of particular clinical settings.

✳   ✳   ✳   ✳

Psychiatric Disorders

Lisa J. Merlo and Nina Gobat

Psychiatric disorders, by definition, cause significant distress and impairment, and symptoms frequently first appear during childhood, adolescence, or young adulthood. Though early treatment can limit the negative consequences of psychiatric disorders and improve current and future functioning, many young people are hesitant to accept their diagnosis or participate in treatment. Other chapters in this volume address externalizing, or "acting-out," behavior problems and eating disorders. Thus, the current chapter focuses on internalizing disorders (i.e., anxiety and depression) and psychotic disorders. Many young people who suffer from anxiety, depression, or psychosis face a range of motivational struggles, both in managing their symptoms and in managing their everyday lives. Therefore, this chapter focuses on ways of integrating MI with other evidence-based treatment approaches in order to maximize positive outcome.

INTERNALIZING DISORDERS

Scope of the Problem

Internalizing disorders are among the most common psychiatric conditions exhibited by youth. They are associated with mood disturbance, worries, behavioral avoidance, and safety rituals, which can lead to significant functional impairment at home, school, and with peers (American Psychiatric Association, 2000). CBT (with or without concurrent pharmacotherapy) is the first-line treatment option for youth with depression or anxiety. However, CBT does not help all young people, and it is noteworthy that a relatively large number of patients do not respond to treatment in a clinically significant manner.

Why MI?

Though most practice guidelines recommend CBT for youth with internalizing disorders, lack of patient motivation and low participation in treatment can negatively impact treatment response (e.g., March, Franklin, Nelson, & Foa, 2001). Thus, you can use MI with your young patients to encourage optimal engagement in CBT-based treatment for internalizing disorders. Indeed, previous research has demonstrated that MI may be most useful when combined with other treatments (Burke, Arkowitz, & Menchola, 2003; Hettema et al., 2005).

For example, the recommended treatment for anxiety disorders (i.e., CBT with exposure and response prevention) can be particularly challenging to young people, due to the requirement that patients engage in exposure exercises (i.e., face their fears). Patients need significant motivation and confidence to voluntarily place themselves in these anxiety-provoking situations, so some of your key tasks as the therapist are: (1) to increase your patient's assessment of the *importance* of completing therapy tasks, and 2) to support your patient's *self-efficacy* regarding his or her ability to be successful.

Similarly, research with adults with obsessive–compulsive disorder (OCD) showed that fears about the potential consequences of symptom reduction can lead to treatment refusal or premature termination (Purdon, Rowa, & Antony, 2004). Among young people, clinical experience suggests that many feel their anxiety symptoms keep them safer or make them "better" in some way. Many also report experiencing secondary gain as a result of their anxiety symptoms. For example, a young person may acknowledge that her disorder provides her with extra attention, control over her family, decreased expectations for completion of chores, an excuse to fail, and "special" status compared to peers. As a result, your patients may feel ambivalent about receiving treatment because they are aware of potential negative consequences to eliminating their symptoms.

You can increase your young patients' motivation for treatment by helping them identify potential benefits of treatment success. For example, teens with internalizing disorders often acknowledge that their symptoms cause a multitude of problems in their lives, including sadness and isolation, excessive worry, wasted time, missed activities, family conflict, frequent "meltdowns," poor school attendance/performance, sleep disturbance, a messy living environment, increased frustration, and/or an inability to take family vacations. Exploring both sides of their experience living with a psychiatric disorder can help to resolve ambivalence about treatment and increase perceptions about the importance of change.

> PRACTITIONER: How might your life be better if your depressive symptoms were under control?

> YOUNG PERSON: Well, I'm sick of feeling this way. I never want to do anything anymore, and some days I can barely get out of bed. Even my friends are starting to get annoyed with me. But I don't have the energy to change. It's too hard.

> PRACTITIONER: You aren't sure what you can do, but you'd like things to be different so that you will feel better again.

> YOUNG PERSON: Yeah, I just wish it wasn't so much work.

> PRACTITIONER: Making *small* changes to improve your mood would be easier for you right now.

MI Spirit and Strategies

MI is based, in part, on the belief that patients are more likely to make a lasting behavioral change if they personally identify and voice their desire, ability, reasons, and needs for making the change (Miller & Rollnick, 2002). However, many young people are referred for therapy by their parents or teachers and have not personally chosen to attend treatment. As a result, rather than adopting an aggressive approach and confronting the young person about the need for treatment, you should elicit the patients' own views regarding their symptoms, as well as their beliefs about the positive and negative consequences of overcoming their disorder. During sessions, you work with the young person to: (1) evaluate the pros and cons of participating in therapy and eliminating symptoms, (2) increase confidence in his or her ability to successfully complete therapy tasks, and (3) prepare for the positive and negative consequences of participation in treatment.

To facilitate this process, it is helpful to begin your session with a structuring statement, followed by an open-ended question for the patient. For example, "Everyone has different experiences and different reasons for coming here. I'd like to know more about your experiences so that I can be most helpful to you in working toward your goals. Tell me a little about how your symptoms are impacting your life." Following up with OARS skills, and utilizing techniques such as expressing empathy and avoiding argumentation, will facilitate rapport-building and strengthen the therapeutic relationship, thus allowing the young person to engage more fully in treatment. In addition, your efforts to support self-efficacy are extremely important when guiding young people through difficult therapy tasks. For example, consider the case of a young person who wanted to avoid completing a difficult exposure exercise:

YOUNG PERSON: I'm not going to touch the toilet seat! That is disgusting! Why would I touch the toilet seat? It's not like people walk around touching toilet seats . . .

PRACTITIONER: You can't imagine any way this would help you overcome your fears.

YOUNG PERSON: Well, I get the point . . . I know it could help, but I don't see any reason why I need to be able to touch a toilet seat. Who does that?

PRACTITIONER: The other exposures were useful because you learned you could successfully do things that you were scared to do before. But it's not worth it to you to prove you could do this too.

YOUNG PERSON: I know I could do it if I wanted to. I just don't want to.

PRACTITIONER: You're confident you could be successful.

In other situations, developing discrepancy, by reviewing how symptoms create a barrier to the patient's aspirations, can be used to guide the patient toward behavior change (e.g., "How does your social anxiety get in the way of your goal of attending the prom?"). Similarly, rolling with resistance, by reflecting/clarifying the patient's fears rather than forcing him or her to engage in a therapy task prematurely, can minimize opposition to your treatment goals or methods (e.g., "It sounds like you don't feel confident that relaxation strategies can help when you start to panic. What concerns do you have about this?").

Working collaboratively with the patient to identify short-term and long-term treatment goals, evaluate potential barriers, and develop a plan of action, may be particularly helpful when reviewing your approach to treatment, planning for between-session "homework" assignments, and looking forward at the termination of formal treatment. In general, you should encourage the young person to take responsibility for his or her own psychological well-being and to set reasonable mini-goals to be reviewed at each session. In doing so, you allow the young person to assume a greater personal investment in his or her treatment. This typically helps to lessen noncompliance, both during and between therapy sessions.

Research Implications

Research studies among adults with generalized anxiety disorder (Westra, Arkowitz, & Dozois, 2008), social anxiety disorder (Buckner & Schmidt, 2008), mixed anxiety/depression (Westra, 2004), and OCD (Maltby & Tolin, 2005) have shown that using MI as part of a pretreatment intervention can encourage CBT acceptance and improve treatment outcome. In addition, one study comparing MI + CBT to psychoeducation + CBT for youth with OCD demonstrated faster treatment gains among the MI + CBT group (Merlo et al., 2010). Given these promising preliminary results, more research is needed to assess the efficacy of incorporating MI-based interventions into treatment for internalizing disorders among young people. In addition, separate randomized studies with large samples are needed for each of the internalizing disorders, and questions regarding the optimal dose and timing of MI need to be answered.

In sum, adding MI to psychotherapeutic treatments for internalizing disorders (e.g., CBT) provides you an important and exciting opportunity to improve rapport with your young patients, encourage active treatment participation, and decrease the likelihood of premature termination.

PSYCHOTIC DISORDERS

Scope of the Problem

According to the World Health Organization (WHO), the cost and burden of psychosis is exceeded only by quadriplegia and dementia (WHO, 2001). Psychotic disorders, the most common of which is schizophrenia, are characterized by cognitive, perceptual, and emotional distortions. With onset typically occurring in adolescence or early adulthood, the course of these disorders is variable. While some young people achieve full recovery, many experience residual or chronic symptoms. Treatment involves a combination of pharmacological and psychosocial interventions involving both the young person and their family (Rossler, Joachim Salize, Van Os, & Riecher-Rossler, 2005). Early detection and treatment of psychosis have become significant psychiatric goals in management and secondary prevention of these conditions.

Why MI?

Rollnick and colleagues (2008) present a general framework for integrating MI within health and social care delivery by shifting between directing, guiding, and following styles of communication. When a client presents as a risk to himself or others, the *directing* style may be most helpful and a practitioner may adopt an approach such as crisis management. When a client is highly distressed emotionally, a *following* style may be called for in which the practitioner listens empathically to a young person's experience with the sole intention of relieving distress. Skillful *guiding* is most suited to conversations about behavior change, and MI is described as a "refined form of this guiding style" (Rollnick et al., 2008, p. 18). Effective practice results from flexible movement between styles to match the presenting situation.

Treatment of psychosis frequently requires multidisciplinary intervention across multiple symptomatic and functional recovery goals. Skillful MI practice can integrate seamlessly with a number of treatment tasks and approaches. In young people with dual diagnosis this has most often been evident with co-occurring substance dependence disorders (Kavanagh et al., 2004). However, there are other areas where MI may have a valuable role. In early phases of treatment, when rapport-building promotes service engagement, MI can help patients resolve their ambivalence about accepting help (Martino, Carroll, O'Malley, & Rounsaville, 2000). Equally, when young people consider accepting more specific interventions such as CBT, integration of MI can promote better outcomes (Barrowclough et al., 2001). MI can be used to improve treatment adherence (Swanson, Pantalon, & Cohen, 1999) and, despite limited research focusing on this area, MI can also be used in self-management discussions (e.g., relapse prevention work) or to support other recovery goals (e.g., vocational aspirations).

MI Spirit and Techniques

Clinical experience suggests that young people with psychosis often feel neglected and disempowered. The spirit of MI emphasizes a helping relationship characterized by collaboration, autonomy support, and evocation. The emphasis on eliciting personal motivation for change, valuing strengths and aspirations, and maintaining a hopeful attitude toward change provides a solid platform for work focused on recovery from psychosis.

Modifications to MI skills may be necessary to accommodate psychotic symptoms and cognitive impairments (Martino, Carroll, Kostas, Perkins, & Rounsaville, 2002). For example, when young people present with disorganized or delusional thinking, the practitioner must reorient the conversation to reality. Keeping language simple and using open-ended questions, frequent simple reflections, and summaries can help to ground the content of the discussion in reality:

YOUNG PERSON: The voices are vices and she knows that, man.

PRACTITIONER: You've been hearing the voices again and it's upsetting you.

YOUNG PERSON: Big time, big time.

PRACTITIONER: Very upsetting.

YOUNG PERSON: Yeah, big time.

When a young person presents with negative symptoms, such as poverty of speech or difficulty making decisions, it can be helpful to use visual aids to stimulate conversation (e.g., a visual agenda-setting chart or decisional balance sheet). Providing sufficient time for the young person to respond is important, and you may find that with these patients, you must speak more than is usually suggested in an MI session.

The need to work across multiple treatment and recovery goals presents a challenge when using MI with this patient group. An agenda-setting strategy is helpful here, as you can identify and strengthen change talk only after a change goal has been identified. Through listening to a young person's narrative, you will elicit a shared agenda of treatment priorities. Thus, one benefit of this strategy is that you can raise potentially contentious topics early on in treatment in a nonthreatening manner, while ensuring that the young person retains a sense of control over the treatment process. Including discussion of the young person's strengths and aspirations develops discrepancy and can enhance motivation to address specific treatment goals. Documenting these priorities visually can help both you and your patient to identify the links between them.

> YOUNG PERSON: *(speaking about her past work experiences)* My head wouldn't work properly so I couldn't carry on.
>
> PRACTITIONER: You were having trouble concentrating.
>
> YOUNG PERSON: Yes, I kept making mistakes.
>
> PRACTITIONER: I know we are talking now about things in this circle *(indicates "work" on the agenda-setting chart)*. And I wonder what was going on in this circle at that time *(indicates "cannabis" on the chart)*?
>
> YOUNG PERSON: Well I was smoking every day then.

As treatment progresses and the therapeutic relationship strengthens, the young person's readiness to address specific change goals is enhanced. Exploration and resolution of ambivalence remain central foci in the therapeutic process.

Research Implications

Modifications to MI for clients with dual diagnosis were developed primarily through work with adults (Martino et al., 2002), as was work integrating MI with CBT (Barrowclough et al., 2001). There is considerable need for research to develop innovative interventions incorporating MI with young people, and for well-designed trials to evaluate them. Despite MI's potential for integrating with a number of treatment approaches in early psychosis, only a limited number of trials have examined its effectiveness. Future research should examine the potential to integrate MI with other approaches in areas such as vocational support and family intervention.

Although the clinical research supporting the use of MI as an adjunct to other psychosocial interventions for young people with psychiatric disorders is in its infancy, preliminary data and clinical experience suggest great potential for its use. Young people suffering from internalizing and/or psychotic disorders may in particular be likely to benefit from MI-guided interventions, owing to the specific challenges inherent to treatment of these disorders.

CHAPTER 15

✳   ✳   ✳   ✳

Eating Disorders

Janet Treasure, Carolina López, and Pam Macdonald

SCOPE OF THE PROBLEM

Eating disorders (EDs) include anorexia nervosa (AN), bulimia nervosa (BN), and eating disorders not otherwise specified (EDNOS). Symptoms include over- or undereating and extreme behaviors related to weight control associated with a significant impairment of psychosocial and physical health. EDs affect mainly young people, with the highest incidence in females between 10 and 19 years old (Currin, Schmidt, Treasure, & Jick, 2005). In terms of prognosis, barely half of all sufferers reach full recovery (Lowe, Zipfel, Buchholz, Dupont, Reas, & Herzog, 2001).

In cases where the course is chronic, the ED can lead to devastating psychosocial and physical consequences with high disability and burden for the sufferer (Steinhausen, 2002, 2009) and their families (Treasure et al., 2005; Whitney & Eisler, 2005; Whitney, Haigh, Weinman, & Treasure, 2007). EDs have the highest rate of mortality linked to a psychiatric disorder because of medical complications and suicide (Harris & Barraclough, 1998). The severe, recurrent course and high level of physical complications associated with EDs also involves an important economic cost for families and the public health care system (Office of Health Economics, 1994; Striegel-Moore et al., 2007).

WHY MI?

Why MI with Sufferers?

A key aspect of AN is that the individual herself does not recognize she has a problem. As one recovered patient said, "I was in love with my anorexia." Their presentation to services, therefore, often involves a degree of coercion from family members, tutors, or occupational health physicians. Consequently, they are not ready to modify their behavior (Blake, Turnbull, & Treasure, 1997). In other forms of ED, sufferers are more willing to change and recognize some aspects of the illness as a problem. However, solving the ambivalence to recover is still a challenge. People with BN, for example, often want to have some symptoms removed (e.g., binges) but are unwilling to tolerate a normal weight.

The MI model has been increasingly utilized in the field of EDs, building on existing assessment and treatment procedures. Some modifications to the standard MI model, however, are required depending on the ED subtype. Many people with AN lack full capacity to make autonomous decisions, either because they are too young or because they are too debilitated by starvation. Nevertheless, you can still work with the spirit of MI, even though the need to have some form of nourishment is a nonnegotiable fact of life. A module of MET with biological and psychological feedback was developed (Treasure & Ward, 1997) and found to be a useful tool in engaging patients with AN (Feld, Woodside, Kaplan, Olmsted, & Carter, 2001; Gowers, Smyth, & Shore, 2004).

MI also is effective in treating adolescents with BN (National Institute for Clinical Excellence, 2004; Schmidt et al., 2007). Sufferers with BN are more likely to be contemplating change as they struggle in the binge-purge cycle. MI allows you to work with these individuals, helping them to explore the ambivalence and resistance to leave the control and/or overcompensatory behaviors (Treasure & Schmidt, 2008).

Why MI with Families of Sufferers?

People with AN are usually dependent on their families either because of their age or because of the severity of their illness. In the United Kingdom, the National Institute for Health and Clinical Excellence (NICE, 2004) guidelines recommended that most people with AN should be managed on an outpatient basis, a policy that places primary responsibility for care on family members. Eating disorder symptoms and the associated high medical risk have profound social ramifications, especially within the family. Caregivers often report lacking the skills and resources required to care for their offspring (Haigh & Treasure, 2003; Treasure et al., 2001). Consequently, the manner in which the family attempts to *reduce* the symptoms often inadvertently plays a role in maintaining or aggravating the problems (Treasure et al., 2008). MI has also proved a useful tool in working with families in many ways. It has helped to model communication skills that both address symptom management and help families change attitudes and behaviors that serve to maintain the disorder.

MI SPIRIT AND STRATEGIES

Using MI with Sufferers

Although a key target problem in people with EDs is eating, this represents only the tip of the iceberg in terms of the difficulties that need to be addressed. Maladaptive emotional regulation strategies, social disconnection, and characteristics of thinking styles are all interim targets that you can work on collaboratively with the young person in contemplating the pros and cons of change. MI addresses each of these domains in combination with motivational and nonthreatening feedback (Emmons & Rollnick, 2001; Miller & Rollnick, 2002).

Thus, in addition to feedback about the medical and nutritional consequences of an ED, you can include personalized feedback on any relevant trait involved in the general assessment. This allows increasing reflection on the predisposing factors/consequences of ED and their role in the sufferer's present lifestyle.

For example, you could incorporate MI to translate cognitive assessment addressing thinking styles into a motivational enhancement module (López, Tchanturia, Stahl, & Treasure, 2008). Thinking styles include cognitive rigidity—for example, difficulties with set-shifting (Roberts et al., 2007) and a narrow focus of vision—for example, weak coherence (López et al., 2008). These contribute to the obsessive–compulsive personality disorder (OCPD) form of the ED phenotype. OCPD is a marker of poor prognosis (Crane, Roberts, & Treasure, 2007) and part of the key maintaining factors of AN (Schmidt & Treasure, 2006).

The following is an excerpt of motivational feedback addressing thinking styles.

> PRACTITIONER: These results suggest that you are somebody who can really grasp details, say, more than the normative population. (Normative Feedback) If we make an analogy with a zoom lens, then, you have the tendency to zoom in on the minute details of life more than somebody who sees the bigger picture. (Generalizing Test Results into Normal Life). I'd be interested in learning how you view this. How would either yourself or other people comment on this observation? (Open Question)

YOUNG PERSON: Yes, I did find that task quite easy . . . I guess I'm quite detailed when I am doing something in my day-to-day life.

PRACTITIONER: Sometimes people with detail can be very good at being tone perfect, or noticing flavors and tastes . . . What type of details would you say you pick up on? (Asking How Details Manifest in Perceptions)

YOUNG PERSON: Yes, I can always tell say if someone has changed something . . . like, for example, when my mother has cleaned my room. I insist on everything being in the same order.

PRACTITIONER: So you really have an eye for that degree of detail. What is helpful about this approach? What's not so great about it? (Analyzing Pros and Cons)

YOUNG PERSON: I think it is quite good to be like that because you don't want to be scrappy, don't want to be messy. I do like things to be perfect . . . probably I do tend to get quite annoyed with people, like with my mother if she has moved things.

PRACTITIONER: So in some ways, other people's standards are not the same as yours and that can cause you a bit of friction. (Complex Reflection)

YOUNG PERSON: Yeah . . . yeah . . .

PRACTITIONER: You've described a situation at home where attention to detail can cause you distress. What scenarios outside the home have proven difficult for you in the past? (Open Question)

YOUNG PERSON: Well . . . If I'm working in a group or something at university or if people are a bit lazy, it really annoys me . . . I suppose I've got too high standards . . . (Acknowledging Problem)

PRACTITIONER: So you can be a bit intolerant of other people not being as . . . *(both laughing)* . . . What problems has this caused? (Exploring the Negative with Open Question)

YOUNG PERSON: Yeah . . . probably I am bossy in a group situation . . . This may annoy other people.

PRACTITIONER: So on the one hand, you can produce high standard work, but on the other hand, working with others who perhaps don't share the same high standards can sometimes cause a bit of friction. (Double-Sided Reflection) Research has shown that this tendency for perfection is common in people with eating disorders. (Relating Detail to Eating Symptoms + Giving Information)

YOUNG PERSON: Yeah, I suppose I do fixate on details . . . in some parts of my body, what I see when I look at myself is just not up to standards and it's probably different to what other people see. It's like when I go to the gym—it's important for me to train harder than others. Trouble is I usually don't feel any better for it! (Acknowledging the Problem).

Further work to develop modules that give feedback about the key emotional, interpersonal and social domains associated with avoidant or more borderline personality traits are in progress (Treasure, 2007; Treasure, Tchanturia, & Schmidt, 2005).

MI with Families of Sufferers

Research suggests that the interpersonal impact of eating disorders is a key maintaining factor (Schmidt & Treasure, 2006). Symptoms of an ED are intrusive, antisocial, anxiety provoking, and frustrating. All semblance of normality disappears, social life evaporates, future plans are put on hold, and interactions around food increasingly dominate all family relationships.

Consequently, it is understandable that responses are often the source of hostile confrontations with family members. Unfortunately, this type of response alienates the individual, who retreats further into ED behaviors, and families acknowledge they need help and skills to manage these behaviors (Haigh & Treasure, 2003).

An excerpt from a typical coaching session working to promote more adaptive communication follows (intervention based in MI techniques are in brackets):

CAREGIVER: I'm going to see her this weekend, so we'll have a chance to talk . . . the trouble though is that I want to get it all out because it's my only opportunity to . . . then of course it all goes horribly wrong.

COACH: You recognize that your anxiety and drive to deliver advice may not be helpful. What's the outcome? (Complex Reflection + Open Question)

CAREGIVER: Oh, she'll just get stressed out by it and then we end up not talking about anything.

COACH: Sounds like it's not working for either of you . . . How can you experiment with different forms of communication that could perhaps alter the outcome? (Complex Reflection + Open Question)

CAREGIVER: I don't know really. I've just got to measure it . . . or think about it beforehand and make sure that if there is an opportunity to sit and talk but just try and see if she'll say something rather than try to push on with the bits I want to talk about.

COACH: I think you are probably correct planning out what would be the best way to get her thinking and talking about change, rather than her defending herself from you talking about why she must change. This is a strategy that research suggests is best for situations when people are in two minds about change. You recognize that your usual way makes things worse if anything. (Affirmation + Giving Information + Complex Reflection)

CAREGIVER: It just gets you full of anxiety and it doesn't help because you do end up blurting out lots of stuff.

COACH: It is hard to be strategic and reflective when you are anxious. (Complex Reflection)

CAREGIVER: Other people say I'm a patient person but . . . it doesn't feel like it—I tend to be very impatient.

COACH: One of your strengths is your patience. If you could play to this strength in your communication about the eating disorder, it might make your meeting on Sunday more positive and less stressful. What is the bigger picture of what you want her to get out of it? (MI-Adherent Response + Open Question)

CAREGIVER: That she does want to get better, that she's got a plan and that I . . . without pushing and doing it for her . . . that she can actually sort things out for herself. I just need to feel more confident and give her the space without insinuating "I know better." I must try not to be too pushy about things . . . just have a little conversation and she can tell me what she's been doing.

RESEARCH IMPLICATIONS

Research on MI with Sufferers

The techniques of MI have been used in many forms of therapeutic interventions for people with ED.

In sufferers, MI has been used as a pretherapy intervention in three studies (Dunn, Neighbors, & Larimer, 2006; Feld et al., 2001; Wade, Frayne, Edwards, Robertson, & Gilchrist, 2009), in a form of personalized feedback in two studies (López, Roberts, Tchanturia, & Treasure, 2008; Schmidt et al., 2006), as motivational enhancement therapy in four studies (Cassin, von Ranson, Heng, Brar, & Wojtowicz, 2008; Dean, Touyz, Rieger, & Thornton, 2008; Feld et al., 2001; Treasure et al., 1999), and as a component of a more complex intervention combined with CBT (Gowers et al., 2004, 2007; Schmidt et al., 2007). Only two of these studies have included exclusively adolescent participants (Gowers et al., 2007; Schmidt et al., 2007).

These studies have consistently demonstrated that MI techniques (in form of MI or MET) improve motivation, confidence, and readiness to change in the ED population (Cassin et al. 2008; Dean et al., 2008; Wade et al., 2009). The effects of MI and MET have also been seen to reduce ED and other psychiatric symptoms. MI and MET, for instance, have been shown to improve the abstinence rate from bingeing in BED (Cassin et al., 2008; Dunn et al., 2006) and helped to decrease depressive symptoms and improve self-esteem in patients with diverse EDs (Field et al., 2001). MET has also been found to be as effective as CBT (Treasure et al., 1999) and more efficient (faster and with lower costs) than family therapy in reducing bulimic symptoms (Schmidt et al., 2007). Furthermore, MET has been successful in promoting treatment continuation in inpatients with ED (Dean et al., 2008). However, it failed to reduce dropouts and to enhance moving into the action phase in outpatients with BN (Treasure et al., 1999).

One of the largest studies in adolescents, and one with the most robust and high-quality design that used MI in combination with CBT (including multimodal and parental feedback), found the level of motivation improved after the initial MI session (Gowers et al., 2007). Interestingly, this intervention was found to be a more cost-effective treatment than either of the more standard forms of adolescent inpatient or outpatient care.

Personalized feedback, one component of MET, has been shown to increase symptom reduction in BN and EDNOS in addition to self-help CBT (Schmidt et al., 2006). In a pilot study, we assessed the effect of a motivational module of personalized feedback as part of the Maudsley individual therapy intervention in outpatients with diverse EDs displaying either cognitive rigidity or extreme attention to detail. Motivational feedback was found to be acceptable and associated with a reduction of perfectionism. In some cases, the reduction in these behaviors generalized to eating behaviors, leading to improvements in BMI, in those with AN (López, 2008). In summary, results suggest that MI techniques are useful in the management of EDs.

Research on MI with Families of Sufferers

As with sufferers, MI has been shown to be an effective intervention for reducing maladaptive interpersonal responses to the symptoms within the family (Sepulveda, López, Macdonald, et al., 2008; Sepulveda, López, Todd, et al., 2008; Treasure, Sepulveda, et al., 2007). Workshops were used to teach families the basic MI skills and to explain the concept of readiness to change, as a way of improving communication as well as reducing expressed emotion, anxiety, and burden (Sepulveda, López, Todd, et al., 2008). Although current research implies the acceptability and feasibility of using MI in working with caregivers, more work is required to identify the most appropriate method of delivery of such an intervention, as well as the extent to which it influences the well-being of the sufferer on his or her path to recovery.

Modifications are presently being implemented into current projects. The number of coaching sessions with caregivers, for example, has been increased. More frequent training and monitoring of coaches' use of MI techniques is taking place, with coaches using the Motivational Interviewing Treatment Integrity (MITI) scales as a self-monitoring tool. Finally, assessments of the sufferers' accounts are being closely monitored for any changes in family dynamics, both positive and negative, upon participation of their caregivers in skills training interventions.

Finally, more research into MI and MET in eating disorders is needed to better understand the role of these interventions in the treatment of adolescents with EDs (in addition to standard treatment, pretreatment, stand-alone therapy, etc.).

ACKNOWLEDGMENTS

This work was part of the ARIADNE program (Applied Research into Anorexia Nervosa and Not Otherwise Specified Eating Disorders), funded by a Department of Health NIHR Program Grant for Applied Research (Reference no. RP-PG-0606-1043) to U. Schmidt, J. Treasure, K. Tchanturia, H. Startup, S. Ringwood, S. Landau, M. Grover, I. Eisler, I. Campbell, J. Beecham, M. Allen, and G. Wolff. The views expressed herein are not necessarily those of DH/NIHR.

CHAPTER 16

✳   ✳   ✳   ✳

Obesity in Minorities

Donna Spruijt-Metz, Elizabeth Barnett, Jaimie Davis,
and Ken Resnicow

SCOPE OF THE PROBLEM

Pediatric obesity has emerged as a major health problem in the United States and globally. In the United States, between 2003 and 2006, 18% of adolescents ages 12–19 years were at or above the 95th percentile of gender- and age-specific body mass index (BMI), and 34% of this age group were above the 85th percentile (Kuczmarski, Ogden, Guo, et al., 2002; Ogden, Carroll, & Flegal, 2008). Obesity rates are substantially higher among African American youth (30% ≥ 95th percentile, 38% ≥ 85th BMI percentile) and Hispanic youth (21% ≥ 95th percentile, 39% ≥ 85th percentile) than their European American counterparts. These health disparities place minority children at disproportionate risk for type 2 diabetes (Narayan, Boyle, Thompson, Sorensen, & Williamson, 2003), metabolic syndrome, some cancers, and a host of other obesity-related diseases. In 1997, the World Health Organization (WHO; 1997) recognized that obesity is a global epidemic, and it has continued to worsen. The WHO's latest projections indicate that globally, approximately 1.6 billion adults (age 15+) are overweight; at least 400 million adults are obese. The WHO projects that by 2015, approximately 2.3 billion adults will be overweight and more than 700 million will be obese. At least 20 million children under the age of 5 years are overweight globally (WHO, 2005).

The psychosocial risks of pediatric overweight are also substantial. Overweight youth are often stigmatized (Kimm et al., 1997; Tiggemann & Anesbury, 2000) as having negative personality characteristics such as cheating, laziness, sloppiness, lying, meanness, and being ugly, dirty, and stupid (Lobstein, Baur, & Uauy, 2004). Overweight and obese children have fewer friends (Strauss & Pollack, 2003) and may grow up to have lower education, income, and likelihood of marriage compared with their thinner counterparts (Gortmaker, Must, Perrin, Sobol, & Dietz, 1993). Obese youth experience discrimination throughout their lives, up to and including gaining admission to college (Lobstein et al., 2004). Finally, overweight has been associated with increased experiences of anxiety, depression, suicidal thoughts, body dissatisfaction, and hopelessness (Lobstein et al., 2004).

Although obesity has a genetic component, it is predominantly caused by behavior, in particular physical inactivity and poor diet. A profound decline in physical activity occurs during early adolescence (Goran, Reynolds, & Lindquist, 1999), particularly in minority populations (Gordon-Larsen, Adair, & Popkin, 2002; Spruijt-Metz, Nguyen-Michel, Goran, Chou, & Huang, 2008; Troiano et al., 2008). As children move into adolescence, the quality of their diet deteriorates, with less intake of fruits and vegetables and more intake of energy-dense, processed foods (Spruijt-Metz, 1999; Taveras et al., 2005). Obesity and obesity-related behaviors such as inactivity and poor diet tend to persist into adulthood and increase the risk of obesity-related conditions later in life (Goran, 2001).

WHY MI?

Pediatric health care practitioners report low confidence in their ability to counsel overweight youth, and they also question the efficacy of behavioral counseling (Kolagotla & Adams, 2004; Perrin, Flower, Garrett, & Ammerman, 2005; Story, et al., 2002). In one study (Kolagotla & Adams, 2004), for example, only 30% of pediatricians felt their efficacy for obesity counseling was good to excellent and only 10% felt that obesity counseling was effective (Kolagotla & Adams, 2004). In another study (Jelalian, Boergers, Alday, & Frank, 2003), only 26% of pediatricians felt "quite" to "extremely" competent to counsel overweight youth and only 37% felt "quite" to "extremely" comfortable providing such treatment (Jelalian et al., 2003). Almost 80% of pediatricians reported feeling "very frustrated" treating pediatric obesity (Jelalian et al., 2003). Low practitioner confidence in their skills and perceptions of treatment futility appear in part to stem from frustration over what they perceive as low parent motivation and poor behavioral adherence (Kolagotla & Adams, 2004; Story et al., 2002) on the part of parents and their children. Perceived patient indifference likely decreases practitioner efficacy as well as perceived treatment utility, which act synergistically to discourage practitioners from attempting to intervene. Importantly, these factors appear to be even more cogent inhibitors than lack of time or reimbursement, and they may be more amenable to intervention. Yet, despite low confidence in their counseling skills, pediatricians and dieticians are interested in improving their behavioral skills (Perrin et al., 2005; Story et al., 2002). MI may address both clinician efficacy and treatment effectiveness in weight-loss counseling.

MI SPIRIT AND STRATEGIES

The experiences using specific MI strategies described in the following sections were accrued from five studies, some ongoing and others completed: (1) *Go Girls* (Resnicow, Taylor, & Baskin, 2005), a church-based nutrition and physical activity program designed for overweight African American adolescent females; (2) *Office-Based Motivational Interviewing to Prevent Childhood Obesity Pilot* (Schwartz et al., 2007), which was designed to test the feasibility and potential efficacy of using MI to reduce childhood obesity in office-based settings; (3) *BMI² Brief Motivational Interviewing to Reduce BMI*, based on the pilot study described above and currently under way; and (4–5) *Strength and Nutrition Outcomes for Latino Adolescents (SANOLA)* and *Strength Training and Nutritional Development for African American Youth (STAND)*, two 16-week diet and physical activity programs that included individual and group MI and were tailored specifically for overweight Latino (SANO) or African American (STAND) adolescents (= 85th BMI percentile, 15.5 ± 1.0 years) (Davis, Kelly, et al., 2009; Davis, Tung, et al., 2009).

Overcoming Environmental Barriers to Change

Young clients often cite environmental factors as reasons that change is difficult. They report that the temptation of fast food is everywhere, that the way their family cooks is a problem, that there is no place to play/exercise in the neighborhood or at school, and finally that due to unsafe communities they opt to stay indoors. If you are involved as a practitioner, you may have expertise in nutrition, exercise, or both that might be useful for the client. In this case, use of a combination of elicit–provide–elicit and complex reflections can be used to provide information and check on how the client receives that information. Such tools as the readiness ruler or values card sort can be used to examine motivation and willingness to change behavior given the new information. Reflective listening and positive affirmations help you to establish a supportive climate for young people, to encourage them to express their own reasons for and against change, and to explore how their current behavior or health status affects their ability to achieve their personal goals. You can juxtapose perceived environmental constraints with motivation to change, guiding the client toward devising a solution that will work in his or her own environment.

Dealing with Demand Characteristics, Exaggerations, and Ensuing Distrust

Self-reports about diet and exercise are influenced by social desirability (reporting what they think they should report), demand characteristics (reporting what they think you want to hear), memory limitations, and the tendency for people to delude themselves a bit when they are not happy with their own behavior. Building rapport and trust by staying within the MI spirit and using MI skills is key to creating an atmosphere in which youth feel comfortable enough to disclose their diet and activity behaviors honestly. Content reflections can help to build initial rapport by showing your interest in the basic facts of the client's story. Content reflections usually paraphrase what the client just said without adding content. Our experience with youth is that a few content reflections at the beginning of the first session help to build rapport. However, we recommend use of feeling/meaning reflections or complex reflections as early in the session as is comfortable. Feeling/meaning reflections often take the form of "You are feeling _____," and may also include a statement about why the person feels a certain way. We have found that acknowledging emotions quickly builds rapport (Resnicow & Rollnick, in press).

Because food and activity choices are made almost constantly in daily life, the opportunity for healthy choices is immense. Even after rapport is developed, youth may report isolated good choices they have made, and may neglect to mention the choices they have made that might be less in tune with their goals. This can result in a multitude of problematic dynamics in the helping relationship, such as overly affirming superficial efforts, distrust and possible dismissal of these reports, questioning of veracity, and clients knowingly telling you what they think you want to hear in order to receive affirmation and avoid discomfort caused by reporting status quo behaviors.

MI spirit and strategies establish trust and rapport, which should encourage youth to honestly disclose diet and physical activity behaviors. However, be prepared to respond to frequent reports of "I had a diet soda" or "I only got a small order of fries" or "I've been eating fewer chips." In these cases, you should acknowledge the youth's efforts and then ask him or her to expand on the episode. Some young people are willing to keep food diaries, which can help you to understand their eating patterns. Keeping a food diary can in itself change behavior; however, when youth are not motivated to keep the diary—when it isn't their own idea—they might not keep precise and consistent records. You can get a better picture of diet and physical activity choices being made by acknowledging the youth's efforts using MI adherent techniques such as an affirming reflection (e.g., "You have really made an effort to lower your soda intake"). Reflections can be followed by an open question to elicit fuller details of a situation in which a particular choice might have been made. We have also used a technique called sensory recruitment (using visual, auditory, olfactory, tactile, and kinesthetic senses to help recall specific situations), borrowed from Interactive Guided Imagery^{SM} to help participants to talk about where they were, who they were with, what was helpful and what was difficult about the situation (Weigensberg et al., 2009).

Changing Hats: The Need to Share Knowledge

A common challenge using MI with obese youth is the need to correct misinformation. For instance, if clients report that they have increased their intake of fruits by drinking fruit-flavored soda, an MI consistent approach might be to use the elicit–provide–elicit (see Chapter 3) in order to let them know that fruit-flavored soda does not have the same nutritional benefits as fruit. The counselor first asks about the client's understanding (Elicit) and then with permission, offers to provide some information, noting when necessary that it might be different from what the client currently believes (Provide), and then again the counselor elicits the client's reaction to this new, and in some cases contradictory, information.

Agenda Setting

For some behavioral problems, such as smoking cigarettes, the target tends to be clear: Either a person smokes or a person does not. When dealing with obesity, however, there can be a broad range of behaviors to target (e.g., eating healthy, sedentary time, increasing physical activity, managing stress.)

In addition to determining what to target, the counselor and client can collaboratively decide on how much change is realistic. For instance, does the client want to "quit" eating fast food, "cut back" on fast food, "reduce" fast-food consumption to one time per week, order the most healthful item on the menu once per week, and so on? Choosing a realistic goal can increase success, perceptions of efficacy, and build client rapport. The differences between these targets can be the difference between client hopelessness: "I'll never be able to quit" and confidence: "I can do that. I can cut back to once a week" or "I can order the grilled chicken sandwich instead of the hamburger."

To assist in this process, an agenda-setting card sort can be of assistance. Young people can choose from a multitude of specific potential target behaviors, ranging from eating more fiber, cutting down on fast food, eating fruit, exercising more, walking to school, increasing sleep, or dealing with stress.

The cards listed below were developed for the Los Angeles SANO/STAND project. You should feel free to add or remove topics as you see fit, as well as allowing participants to add their own, more specific, targets if the cards do not contain the change they wish to make.

Agenda-Setting Cards

Eat more fruits	Drink fewer sugary	Eat less school food
Eat more	drinks	Eat less fast food
vegetables	Eat less junk food	Eat smaller portions
Go grocery	Drink more water	Make lunch night
shopping	Eat breakfast	before
Cook more of my	Do more exercise	Take lunch to school
own meals	Skip fewer meals	Eat lunch

Once the young person selects a behavior(s) he or she would like to target, you then ask about the reasons that she or he chose this behavior(s). This is consistent with the MI concept of linking behavior change to underlying values. Use reflections and open questions to explore and thereby deepen participant engagement and motivation, avoiding the temptation to immediately ask questions about how the client can achieve this change. At this point in time, the immediate goal is for both you and the young person to develop a greater understanding of both the advantages and disadvantages of change from the client's perspective, as well as the meaning of change. Prematurely pushing for change can generate reactance from the young person.

Common Motivations and Barriers to Change

When asked, young clients usually report a variety of reasons for wanting to reduce the risks associated with obesity. Their motivation ranges from a family history of disease, disability, amputation, or death due to obesity-related illnesses to their own problems at school such as being teased, or a desire for boyfriends/girlfriends. Despite the poignancy of their desires, many young people also express powerlessness to deal with their fate. Young clients often believe that their weight is biologically determined; they cite being big-boned, having slow metabolism, and/or getting disease due to heredity and not their behavior. In many cases, these ideas represent the beliefs of their families and others suffering from the effects of obesity.

A key MI strategy is to roll with such resistance, in effect agreeing with the client rather than refuting or counter-arguing. An especially powerful strategy in these cases is the amplified negative reflection, whereby the counselor exaggerates the client's beliefs; for example, "you see no role in your behavior . . ." or, "you think it is all genetically determined." By arguing against change, it is possible that the client's negativity "gives out"—or becomes exhausted. In response, the clients may reverse their course and start to argue for change. This type of reflection is not without potential risks and can occasionally backfire. A key issue is to avoid any tone of sarcasm. This type of reflection is particularly useful when clients appear to be stuck in a "yes, but" mindset (Resnicow & McMaster, in press).

Another way to defuse these ideas is to again use elicit–provide–elicit. For instance, after *eliciting* beliefs, you can ask permission to *provide* additional information about for example the genetic basis of weight regulation, or you can reframe client ideas as a way to expand the client's understanding, and then *elicit* reactions to the reframing. Doubled-sided reflections can help reduce *reactance* from clients, as they show that the counselor appreciates the complexity of the situation and is not trying to prematurely push them to change, and they can also move clients from the "yes, but . . ." mindset. For instance, if a participant states that "everyone in my family has diabetes," a reflection might be to offer empathy and opportunity: "You feel like you'll probably get diabetes too, and at the same time, you're thinking about what kind of changes you can make."

MI as a Prelude/Adjunct
to Other Empirically Supported Treatments

Although MI has been established as a useful method for helping individuals overcome resistance and clarify motivation, additional strategies such as behavior therapy or cognitive-behavioral therapy may be indicated once an individual decides to attempt behavior change. MI can be seen as the key strategy in building the reason for change, that is, *why* change, whereas other techniques/modalities can be brought to bear when discussing *how* to change. Thus, MI should perhaps be conceived as a platform for treatment delivery rather than the primary treatment modality. How best to integrate standard cognitive and behavioral weight-loss strategies within an MI framework merits examination.

To this end, Resnicow and Rollnick have recently proposed a three-phase model of MI, adapted from Rollnick, Miller, and Butler (2007, 2008). The three phases—explore, guide, and choose—integrate more action-oriented modalities into the MI consultation. In *exploring*, the primary objective is to elicit the client's story, build rapport through empathy, obtain a behavioral history that includes prior attempts to change, and collaborate with the client to decide what behaviors to address during the session. Key skills here include listening, shared agenda setting, open-ended questions, content, feeling, and double-sided reflections. During the *guiding* phase, the counselor moves the conversation toward the possibility of change. You could elicit change talk by asking the client to consider life with and without change and by building discrepancy between the client's current actions and his or her broader life goals and values. You might choose to end by inviting the client to commit to making a change, for example, "so where does that leave us?" Key strategies used during this phase include 0-to-10 importance/confidence rulers, values clarification, and summarizing. If the client expresses a clear commitment to making a change, the session can move to the *choosing* phase, a discussion of *how* to implement the change. The main objectives in this phase are helping clients identify a goal, choosing an action plan, anticipating barriers, and agreeing on a plan for monitoring and a reinforcement schedule. Key skills for this phase are action reflections, menu building, and goal setting. CBT and other behavioral strategies are woven into the choosing phase.

Additional Considerations for Working with Overweight Youth

The promotion of physical activity and healthy diets in young people is complicated by the consistent exposure to "obesogenic" environments, an exposure that is higher in minority youth. Obesogenic environments offer minimal opportunities and resources for physical activity (Kipke et al., 2007), a host of attractive, inexpensive, and high-calorie foods, a dearth of healthy foods (food deserts) (Lewis et al., 2005), lower frequency of meals eaten together with the family, and high exposure to chronic stress, including crime and disturbed family and social connections (Booth, Pinkston, & Poston, 2005). Motivating youth to change diet and physical activity behaviors in the face of these contextual challenges has proven daunting. However, each of these challenges can be addressed as part of a targeted behavior action plan.

Consider the youth's specific environment and be prepared to deal with such family and cultural issues. When working with minority youth in particular, it is helpful to be familiar with available resources for physical activity in the community or at school as well as with amenities such as easily accessible grocery outlets in the neighborhood. This promotes an understanding of the forces affecting these youth and opens the possibility of offering appropriate suggestions should these seem warranted when using the elicit–provide–elicit framework.

Another major barrier to implementing behavior change is related to culturally specific definitions of attractiveness and ideal body image. African American and Hispanic youth have a larger ideal body type than their white counterparts, and are more likely, when clinically overweight, to still feel attractive (Becker, Yanek, Koffman, & Bronner, 1999; Resnicow et al., 2000). Overweight youth who are comfortable with their size may not see an immediate need to change behavior, regardless of health consequences.

The emphasis of the motivational interview might focus on health-related outcomes, for instance avoiding diabetes or other diseases that overweight youth might see regularly in their family and/or community, exercising to feeling more energetic, or dropping certain foods from their diets to develop self-discipline. However, a key element of MI, and other client-centered approaches to counseling, is that the counselor helps the clients find their unique motivation without attempting to persuade with health information or fear messages. It is important to keep in mind that there are many personal motives—some of which the counselor might not anticipate—for overweight youth to change behaviors, motives that are not necessarily related to their body size or to their health.

Few interventions are available or tailored to meet the needs of African American (Resnicow et al., 2000, 2005) and Hispanic youth (Spruijt-Metz et al., 2008; Spruijt-Metz & Saelens, 2005). Youth who live with violence or poverty often have more fundamental life issues on their mind than their own health. Therefore, flexibility and responsiveness to the youth's concerns are key, and approaching eating and activity patterns within the context of their physical and social environmental can help make the counseling more salient to minority youth.

RESEARCH IMPLICATIONS

MI to prevent and treat pediatric obesity has been used in randomized, controlled multicenter trials (DISC) (Berg-Smith et al., 1999), intensive randomized controlled interventions (SANO) (Davis, Kelly, et al., 2009; Davis, Tung, et al., 2009), doctor/clinician offices (Schwartz et al., 2007), community-based interventions (WATCHIT) (Rudolf et al., 2006), churches (GO GIRLS) (Resnicow et al., 2005), and school settings (NEW MOVES) (Flattum, Friend, Neumark-Sztainer, & Story, 2009). Results from these efforts have been mixed, with the DISC study showing significant changes in diet and metabolic markers, the SANO study showing some significant changes in metabolic health outcomes, WATCHIT significant reductions in BMI, and GO GIRLS no significant changes in main outcomes. At this moment, outcomes from the NEW MOVES study are not yet available.

Several of these studies were pilot studies with small sample sizes. Furthermore, the implementation of MI in each of these interventions was widely divergent, including differences in hours training and supervision of MI providers, who received the sessions (parent, child, or family), session structure, and, importantly, number of sessions. Schwartz and colleagues (2007) tested two different intervention intensities. One group of parents received one MI session, while another received four MI sessions. There was a nonsignificant incremental decrease in the child's BMI with increased number of sessions. However, dropout quadrupled in the intense group as compared to the control group. These important issues of implementation have yet to be fully explored and delineated.

Changing obesity-related behaviors may prove most challenging when parents are also overweight. Moreover, because Hispanic and African Americans experience higher rates of obesity in the United States, minority youth will more likely have overweight parents (Ogden, Yanovski, Carroll, & Flegal, 2007). Depending on the age of the youth, the intervention may occur directly with the parent(s), directly with the young person, or both. Some evidence exists that obese adolescents do not benefit from the involvement of their parents, whereas parent involvement may be beneficial for younger children (Resnicow, 2002). However, it is not known at what age youth and parents should be seen alone versus together. This may differ by race/ethnicity as well. Evidence from SANO (unpublished data) shows that participants had better outcomes when their parents attended more of the education sessions.

The use of MI in minority youth also raises some unique research and practice issues. Although several studies have shown that MI can be useful to modify diet and activity behaviors in African Americans (Resnicow et al., 2002, 2004, 2005; Resnicow, Jackson, Wang, Dudley, & Baranowski, 2001) and Latino youth (Davis, Kelly, et al., 2009; Davis, Tung, et al., 2009), more research is needed to determine whether MI may operate differently with some ethnic groups.

CHAPTER 17

❋　　❋　　❋　　❋

Self-Care for Chronic
Medical Conditions

Sylvie Naar-King and Deborah Ann Ellis

SCOPE OF THE PROBLEM

Many chronic health conditions require a variety of complicated daily tasks to manage the disease. For instance, young people with diabetes must take insulin, keep careful track of carbohydrate intake, test blood glucose levels several times a day, and respond to fluctuations in these levels. Young people with severe asthma typically take controller medications, monitor lung functioning daily, carry an inhaler, and avoid allergens. Historically, the phenomenon of self-care behavior has been described using various terms. Formerly termed "compliance" or "adherence" to medical recommendations, self-care behavior refers to the complex processes a patient and a physician collaboratively agree should be completed to manage the chronic condition. While compliance and adherence imply that the patient must follow a set of rules mandated by an authority figure, self-care refers to the decisions and activities individuals undertake with the intention of limiting the consequences of illness and enhancing health (WHO, 2001). Poor self-care implies that the behaviors the individual has chosen to implement (smoking) or avoid (testing blood sugars) serve to undermine health and result in inadequate management of the chronic condition.

Difficulty following medical treatment recommendations is a common cause of treatment failure in pediatric populations (LaGreca & Shulman,

1995; Milgrom et al., 1996), including diabetes (Morris et al., 1997; Smith, Firth, Bennett, Howard, & Chisholm, 1998), asthma (Weinstein & Faust, 1997), HIV (Naar-King et al., 2006), and cardiac transplant (Dobbels et al., 2005). Illness management skills have been shown to deteriorate in adolescence (Drotar & Ievers, 1994) and are often associated with an increase in other risky behaviors. Most commonly evidenced during adolescence, poor self-care serves specific social and psychological developmental functions (e.g., individuation from the family, seeking acceptance from peers; see Jessor, 1992). Outcomes can be further worsened as a result of the adolescent's cognitive immaturity and/or lack of a future-oriented perspective. This may limit his or her ability to effectively weigh the potential long-term health risks of poor self-care against the immediate gains he or she obtains by avoiding or ignoring necessary health care tasks.

WHY MI?

Studies show that during adolescence, parents tend to decrease involvement and supervision of their teens' daily activities (Laird, Pettit, Bates, & Dodge, 2003; Wysocki et al., 1996). Thus, as adolescents become increasingly responsible for managing their own conditions, internal motivation for self-care becomes critical. Building motivation is especially important as the chronically ill adolescent transitions into the adult health care system. The young person becomes responsible for illness management decisions, yet during this transitional period, disengagement from the medical setting has been shown to increase. One study found that more than half of adolescents with congenital heart defects did not successfully transition into adult services, as evidenced by their failure to attend adult care appointments (Reid, McCrindle, Sananes, & Ritvo, 2004). Similarly, young adults with HIV have been found to be at high risk of missing appointments, which interferes with monitoring immune function and determining the need to begin medications (Ashman, Conviser, & Pounds, 2002).

Research has begun to confirm that motivation to change is related to better self-care both in terms of illness management behaviors (MacDonell et al., 2010) and via increased engagement in health care (Outlaw et al., in press). Finally, studies have also shown self-efficacy to be an important factor in adolescent self-care (Naar-King et al., 2006; Schwarzer & Luszczynsko, 2006). Thus, while self-care behavior is determined by multiple factors across medical and familial systems, increasing the young person's motivation and efficacy for self-care may assist in improving illness management and health outcomes. A final and critical component of illness management is family involvement; factors related to MI with families are addressed in Chapter 20.

MI SPIRIT AND STRATEGIES

The first step in an MI approach to improving self-care in adolescents and young adults with chronic conditions is to ensure that the young person has taken an active role in developing his or her medical treatment plan. An adolescent may be disengaged or be less involved in treatment planning if the treatment team focuses more on parental goals than on the teen. Thus, it is critical for you to understand the context in which the treatment plan was developed, as well as to recognize the importance of including adolescents in the decision-making process to ensure long-term successful illness management as they transition into adulthood. You support adolescent autonomy (Williams, Cox, Kouides, & Deci, 1999) by communicating a valuing of the patient's perspective (e.g., reflecting ambivalence about treatment), minimizing pressures and demands placed on the young person (e.g., asking for permission before providing information) and offering choices wherever possible (e.g., providing a menu of self-care options).

As in all MI interventions, the first step is to establish rapport and elicit patient concerns. The opening statement is especially critical as the young person may perceive the session as "just another medical visit" and expect either to be told what to do or to be treated as simply another youth with inadequate self-care. Alternatively, the young person may be resistant to engaging in behavioral health services when a mental health problem such as depression is not present. The elicit–provide–elicit strategy may be helpful at this early juncture (see Chapter 3). Beginning the session by eliciting the young person's view of why he or she is there can help to identify potential resistance, starting at the onset of treatment. Consider asking, "Tell me some of the reasons you think that someone referred you here?" Then follow with an opening statement, such as: "Our meeting today may be different from other medical visits, in that I am not here to tell you what to do or how to do it. Rather, I want to find out what you might be interested in changing and what might help." For those young persons who are more resistant to a mental health session, consider also statements such as: "This does not have to be a time to talk about psychological problems. Rather, you have difficult choices to make for your health, and this is a place that you can talk over those choices." Then elicit the person's view of this approach.

Because of the multiple behaviors typically involved in illness management, the strategy of agenda setting may be particularly useful after establishing rapport (see Chapter 3). It is important for the practitioner to have enough familiarity with the illness being treated to lay out all the behavior options for discussion and to guide the patient to focus on behaviors that they are not only ready to change but that also might have the greatest impact on health outcomes.

Following these opening strategies, elicit the young person's view of the agreed upon target behavior using OARS. As a result of the serious health consequences that poor self-care behaviors can cause to the young person, the pressure for the practitioner to promote behavior change may be particularly strong. Of the six traps described by Miller and Rollnick (2002), two can be particularly tempting, and practitioners are cautioned to avoid their use. In the first trap, "Premature Focus," the practitioner adheres to a strict agenda for addressing the young person's medical treatment plan and disregards (or ignores) the young person's other, more relevant and pressing concerns (e.g., peer issues, parental conflict). Not only can this unwavering practitioner stance engender the young person's resistance to discuss behavior change, but it also ruptures the therapeutic alliance if the young person feels ignored or not taken seriously.

The sense of urgency practitioners may have about preserving the young person's health may also result in the second common trap, "Taking Sides." The risk of falling into these traps may be especially high when the young person expresses both sides of their ambivalence to make a change. In our experience, it is rare for a young person with a chronic illness to be completely resistant to any medical intervention. For example, often we have heard a young person with HIV state, "I am supposed to take medication to keep my viral load down, but sometimes I just don't feel like it." It is common for the well-intentioned practitioner immediately to take the side of taking medication, responding with a statement such as: "Your viral load is high and if you don't start taking medication your immune system will shut down." Falling into this trap early in the session often creates the opportunity for a young person experiencing ambivalence to argue for reasons not to change, as well as find flaws in the practitioner's logic. For example, a young person may respond, "Well, I am not taking medication now, and my immune system is just fine."

An alternative approach centers on the reflection of ambivalence. For example, an amplified reflection could be, "It seems that you really see no reasons for taking your medication." Your amplification of the ambivalence, paired with a nonargumentative stance, allows the young person to provide his or her own reasons for change and begin to address areas of needed behavioral intervention. For example, reasons to change are communicated with statements such as: "Yes, but the doctor says that if I don't, my virus could grow and be harder to fight off later."

Another approach to avoiding this trap of taking sides is to explore ambivalence more effectively via the elicitation of the pros and cons of behavior change. The "Decisional Balance" strategy allows the practitioner to pave the way toward reinforcing change talk, by addressing the frustrations associated with completing self-care tasks and ending with an analysis of the positive outcomes that may result from change. In our work with young adults with HIV, the most common pros of taking medications were related to controlling illness and living longer. Over 75% of the sample rated this as a very important reason to take medication, supporting the contention that most youth see some benefit in taking medications. The most common cons of taking medication were the side effects. Interestingly, more than 25% of the sample agreed with the statement that "it does not matter if you take your medications because you will die anyway." From an information-processing perspective (see Chapter 2 for details), some young people are less reactive to thoughts about negative consequences of risky behavior because they have a pessimistic perception about leading a long, happy life (Chapin, 2001). Some adolescents feel that bad things will happen regardless of their behavior, and this outlook may be intensified when managing a chronic condition.

Three key strategies to enhance self-efficacy (belief in your ability to follow the treatment plan) and improve response efficacy (belief in the efficacy of your treatment) include: (1) providing individualized feedback of medical tests with a discussion of the relationship of these results to the young person's engagement in self-care behaviors; (2) employing the imagining extremes strategy; and (3) gathering information about prior successes in behavior change. In the discussion of feedback and its utility for effecting change, you offer only facts from the medical tests and allow the young person to interpret the impact of the results on his or her chronic illness. For example, by providing objective feedback regarding the young person's blood glucose levels and collaboratively discussing how the young person's self-care behaviors have an impact on these levels, motivation for self-care may improve.

With the imagining extremes strategy, you elicit from the person his or her imagined worst fears if treatment were to be stopped, along with the best outcomes that might occur if the treatment plan was consistently followed. As managing a given illness often consists of completing several interrelated self-care behaviors, it is often possible to find one area of self-care that the adolescent is managing well. Finally, the you might gather information regarding other health behaviors the person is performing well, even if not directly related to the illness (e.g., getting enough sleep, eating a healthy diet, not smoking), and reflect this strength as evidence of ability for behavior change.

When the young person is ready to make a change, strategies such as the "Menu of Options" and "Giving Information" are also relevant using elicit–provide–elicit (see Chapter 7), but be careful about the limits of your own expertise. Often, referral to the medical team may be most appropriate, and certainly guiding the young person to advocate for his or her own treatment is critically important for long-term success. You must also be cautious about utilizing a harm-reduction model, which suggests that small changes in behavior may be the more appropriate approach to achieving long-term behavioral goals. While some self-care behaviors can be appropriately targeted with this model (e.g., working on testing blood sugar at least once a day if not ready to test several times per day as prescribed), others cannot (e.g., taking less than 100% of HIV medications 90% of the time may have unintended negative consequences by promoting viral resistance). Thus, practitioners should be clear about the medical implications of the young person's goal setting.

RESEARCH IMPLICATIONS

Although several published papers have suggested the relevance of MI for improving self-care in adolescents and young adults (Sindelar et al., 2004), randomized clinical trials are rare. In a multisite randomized trial, Naar-King, Parsons and colleagues (2009) showed that a four-session MI intervention with individualized feedback improved health outcomes in young people living with HIV. Channon and colleagues (2007) found that adolescents with diabetes receiving an average of four MI sessions over 12 months showed significantly greater improvements in average blood glucose level (HbA1c) than adolescents receiving nondirective, supportive counseling. Naar-King, Outlaw and colleagues (2009) reported that young adults receiving two sessions of MI from a peer mentor or from a master's-level clinician improved their attendance at HIV primary care appointments. All three studies had relatively small sample sizes (less than 100 participants), but provide promising initial evidence of the utility of MI in enhancing self-care behaviors. Clearly, further research is needed with larger samples and with other chronic conditions to determine MI's ability to improve motivation and self-efficacy for self-care in adolescents and young adults. Furthermore, given that other factors besides motivation and self-efficacy may be associated with self-care, studies combining MI with other interventions such as cognitive-behavioral skills training or family systems interventions are warranted.

CHAPTER 18

✳   ✳   ✳   ✳

Group Alcohol and Drug Treatment

Elizabeth J. D'Amico, Sarah W. Feldstein Ewing, Brett Engle,
Sarah Hunter, Karen Chan Osilla, and Angela Bryan

SCOPE OF THE PROBLEM

Youth who use alcohol and other drugs (AOD) are at risk of suffering a range of serious consequences (Johnston et al., 2008). For example, adolescents who begin to use alcohol more heavily during the teen years are more likely to report unsafe sex (Yan, Chiu, Stoesen, & Wang, 2007; Zimmer-Gembeck & Helfand, 2008) and delinquent behavior, such as picking fights, stealing, or vandalism (Ellickson & McGuigan, 2000; Ford, 2005; Loeber & Farrington, 2000).

Group work is the most common AOD treatment modality (Rotgers, Morgenstern, & Walters, 2003) especially for adolescents (Flores & Mahon, 1993; Piper & McCallum, 1994) as it is cost-effective (Kaminer, Burleson, & Goldberger, 2002), promotes social support seeking (Piper & McCallum, 1994), and other developmentally salient interpersonal skills (Dies, 2000). Group work is also similar to youths' everyday lives as they are constantly interacting with their peers (Kaminer et al., 2002). It may therefore be a more attractive and less threatening approach than an individual intervention (MacLennan & Dies, 1992; Shechtman, 2002). However, others warn that this modality is not only ineffective but iatrogenic (Dodge, Dishion, & Lansford, 2006). That is, some group interventions increase rather than decrease risk behaviors (Dishion, McCord, & Poulin, 1999). Thus, once a group is formed, group leaders must take steps to monitor and discourage negative peer interactions from counteracting the benefits of the group intervention.

WHY MI?

Despite the probability of risk and consequences related to substance use, most youth do not seek help for AOD use. This may be due to stigma (Corrigan, 2004), concerns about confidentiality (Dubow, Lovko, & Kausch, 1990; Rickwood, Deane, & Wison, 2007), feelings of disconnection from the person implementing the service (D'Amico, 2005), failure to view substance use as problematic (Johnson, Stiffman, Hadley-Ives, & Elze, 2001; Marlatt, Larimer, Baer, & Quigley, 1993), or difficulties articulating the problems associated with their substance use (Feldstein Ewing, Hendrickson, & Payne, 2008). These barriers suggest that intervention efforts focused on reducing adolescent AOD use would benefit from including the following features: (1) presentation of treatment in a developmentally conscious manner, (2) avoidance of procedures that could stigmatize youth, (3) collaborative work with youth to identify harm-reduction strategies, (4) utilization of active, strength-based efforts that enhance positive, prosocial behaviors, and (5) active emphasis on the youth's autonomy to bolster the sense of self-efficacy (Feldstein Ewing, Walters, & Baer, in press).

MI may be ideally suited to address potential barriers when working with adolescent groups because it is inherently collaborative, focusing on achievable approaches for change (Feldstein & Ginsburg, 2007). Described as a "guiding" approach, MI practitioners actively elicit client participation, with the goal of highlighting the youth's ambivalence about a target behavior, drawing out and reinforcing pro-change language and change talk (Miller & Rollnick, 2002).

Often, when at-risk youth are mandated to group programs, the "interventions" are didactic programs, which have low evidence for efficacy (Reyna & Farley, 2006; Tobler, 2000). Moreover, in these settings, youth are frequently told that they need to change and that not doing so will result in more trouble (e.g., "If we find out that you haven't stopped using, we'll report you to probation"). Rarely are youth provided with the opportunity to give voice to why change might be helpful and/or with practical strategies for approaching change efforts.

Studies have suggested that the nonjudgmental, empathic, and collaborative approach of MI makes it ideal for at-risk youth from disadvantaged/marginalized or cultural minority backgrounds (D'Amico, Miles, Stern, & Meredith, 2008; Hettema, Steele, & Miller, 2005). MI allows the client's values, opinions, and arguments for change to be the most valued component of the discussion (Miller, Villanueva, Tonigan, & Cuzmar, 2007). Moreover, MI's guiding approach allows at-risk youth, who may be inherently distrustful of authority, to articulate their frustration with the intervention process without halting the process.

MI approaches are ideal for the group setting, for they naturally initiate group interaction and collaboration, two components integral to achieving positive outcomes (Tobler & Stratton, 1997). Furthermore, many MI principles are consistent with the advocated approaches within the group work literature. For example, social group work theories recognize and build upon group member strengths, as well as use reflections and open questions rather than give instructions or advice (Northen & Kurland, 2001). Indeed, many group work approaches are sensitive to issues of power and authority and emphasize group member autonomy and the supportive role of the group leader (e.g., Malekoff, 2004).

MI SPIRIT AND STRATEGIES

As noted by Feldstein Ewing and colleagues (in press), several important considerations differentiate group from individual MI. They include the (1) more complicated interpersonal dynamics of the group process (e.g., monitoring between-client conversations; group cohesion; peer influence), and (2) varying experiences and needs of the participants (e.g., different substance use experience) that require a simultaneous response to different individual needs (e.g., rolling with the resistance of one youth, while trying to actively maintain the commitment language of another). To address these issues, we next review several recommendations for structuring and tailoring the group.

Structuring the Group

1. Be clear about the reason for holding the group and maintain the focus throughout the group.
2. Keep groups small (i.e., fewer than 9–10 members) and sessions brief (1 hour).
3. Generate the majority of session content from participants.
4. Initiate and maintain a positive and judgment-free atmosphere throughout the group.

Pros and Cons of Continued Use

A discussion of the pros and cons of continued AOD use (Ingersoll, Wagner, & Gharib, 2006) can be a powerful tool in group settings. This involves having youth collaboratively generate examples of the good and "not so good" things that may occur if they continue using AOD or if they decide to stop using AOD. For example, you may initiate exploration like this,

"We know that you guys are smart, and have chosen to use substances for important reasons. Tell me some of the reasons why you like using alcohol." While the creators of MI (Miller & Rollnick, 2002) currently debate the utility of this approach within adult settings (e.g., Miller, 2008), we have found it useful in adolescent groups. First, it provides young people with the sense that they are not foolish; rather, they had several life choices or events that led to their substance use. Second, it can help you to identify areas to target for harm reduction (e.g., if adolescents are using for stress reduction). Third, group exploration of the pros and cons enables youth to give voice to the "not-so-great" aspects of their substance use behavior. Moreover, adolescents are more likely to give credence to negative consequences voiced by peers than negative consequences suggested by group leaders.

Discuss Current and Future Goals

Another useful group MI strategy involves having teens discuss current and future goals (Ingersoll et al., 2006), which can help them explore and develop discrepancy between their behavior and goals. Discussion of goals is important, for this discrepancy is posited to catalyze behavior change within MI (Miller & Rollnick, 2002). For example, the group leader might say to the group, "OK, let's hear where you guys see yourself within a year? What do you see yourself doing in 2 years?; How does being a soccer star fit with heavy marijuana use?"

Establish Group Goals: Problem-Solving Skills and Harm Reduction

Establishing group goals can set the groundwork for building group-generated harm-reduction approaches, such as planning for change using problem-solving skills (Ingersoll et al., 2006). For example, the group leader can ask youth to think about how to plan and prepare for high-risk situations where AOD may be present. They can then discuss in the group if anyone has previously tried these strategies, whether they were successful, if they feel that these strategies have potential to work in these situations, and so on: "Gosh, so one of the things that I'm hearing throughout the group is that lots of you feel like alcohol helps you when things start to get really tough at school. Using alcohol is one way to reduce that stress. What are some other ways that the group has found helpful to reduce school-related stress?" Offering youth the opportunity to generate their own harm-reduction strategies can give the adolescent a strong sense of self-efficacy and dovetails with effective alcohol treatment approaches (Moos, 2007). Group members can spontaneously support one another in making these plans. Discussion can focus on whether the plan is possible, and members can help each other determine whether changes need to be made to ensure the plan will be successful.

Attend to Commitment Statements

Not only is it important that you closely attend to group member statements regarding AOD use (or other target behaviors), but also it is crucial to attend to other group members' responses to these commitment statements (Engle, Macgowan, Wagner, & Amrhein, 2010). This can help you determine whether group members will reduce or increase the target behavior. Also, your empathy may be integral to fostering positive and/or diminishing negative group member language and processes.

RESEARCH IMPLICATIONS

Conducting group work with adolescents presents unique opportunities and challenges. Several recent reviews conclude that group work with at-risk adolescents is generally effective and comparable to individual interventions (e.g., Kaminer, 2005; Vaughn & Howard, 2004; Waldron & Turner, 2008). Research on group interventions with at-risk youth that utilize motivational interviewing, however, is only just emerging (Bailey, Baker, Webster, & Lewin, 2004; Feldstein Ewing et al., in press; Schmiege et al., 2009). While preliminary data supports the use of group MI, below we discuss three recent studies that have begun to more intricately address process, format, and outcomes of group MI with adolescents.

One example of using an MI approach with at-risk youth in a group setting comes from D'Amico, Osilla and Hunter's (in press) work with first-time AOD offenders. In this setting, teens are offered the opportunity to attend a six-session AOD education group as part of a sentence that will allow them to remove the offense from their record. D'Amico and colleagues developed and piloted the six sessions two to three times with groups of adolescents and obtained feedback on the content and style of each session. They used several MI approaches in these sessions, including open-ended questions, discussion of the pros and cons of use, goal setting, problem solving, and teens' willingness and confidence to change their AOD behavior.

Qualitative data were collected at the end of each group session (D'Amico et al., in press). Overall, the data show that the group MI intervention fit well with the teens' developmental stage, was not perceived as stigmatizing, and conveyed the MI concepts well. Specifically, the group MI participants stated that they did not feel like they were being judged, and the group facilitator was empathic: "Like if we said something, no one was saying, 'That's wrong!'; "I liked that no one was judging you"; "She was like really open and nonjudgmental; "She was very cool and open and listened to what we had to say." Consistent with effective MI approaches, teens reported that the sessions were collaborative: "This was better than the other classes where they just talk at you the whole time"; "[I] liked the way [she] asked questions to make people more interested"; "In like some groups, some people don't talk at all. She kind of got everybody involved."

As expected, most of the teens in the groups were at different places in terms of their willingness to change. They acknowledged this difference and liked that the MI focus of the group guided them and that they were not told to change their behavior, which is consistent with MI's focus on building self-efficacy: "A lot of kids want to know how to change. They are asking for help, but don't want to ask [out loud], so seeing it [on a handout] is better than having someone just telling you, 'You have to change, what are you going to do about it!?'"

In another study, Engle and colleagues (2010) analyzed commitment language and related MI process constructs as markers of marijuana use outcomes of 12- to 18-year-olds participating in an 8-week adolescent group treatment. Replicating studies of individual MI sessions with adults (Amrhein, Miller, Yahne, Palmer, & Fulcher, 2003), Engle and colleagues found that commitment language and peer group member responses to commitment language both predicted marijuana use outcomes. "I'm quitting for the summer" and "I'll never stop smoking weed" are examples of positive and negative commitment language utterances, respectively. Positive and negative peer responses to such commitment language included utterances, such as "that's great" or "what a lightweight," as well as laughing or clapping. The language spoken in the group context correlated with group member marijuana use outcomes. Specifically, the more positive and less negative the peer responses, the greater the reduction in marijuana use. Moreover, group leader empathy was associated with more positive commitment language and peer responses to commitment language.

One final example highlighting a potential modality for group MI with at-risk adolescents is the use of a single session of group MI to augment other psychosocial interventions. Similar to findings from the adult literature (Hettema et al., 2005), Bryan and Feldstein Ewing's (2008) preliminary data supports the utility of group MI in an add-on design rather than as a stand-alone intervention. This "augmenting" approach enables a single session of group MI to target treatment engagement or content that would otherwise not be a part of the main psychosocial intervention (e.g., addressing substance use during a sexual risk reduction program (Schmiege et al., 2009). Notably, 3-month outcome data for these youth indicated that adolescents who received the group-MI augmented sexual risk reduction intervention showed greater reduction in sexual risk behavior than adolescents in the control or traditional sexual risk reduction intervention (Schmiege et al., 2009).

These three recent studies highlight the potential for adolescent group MI to engage at-risk youth and initiate contemplation of behavior change. However, further work is needed in several areas. First, it is important to examine both short- and long-term outcomes of group MI on adolescents' AOD use. In addition, it will be important to assess how certain factors, including commitment language and peer responses during the group (i.e., cohesiveness, etc.), affect behavioral outcomes.

Furthermore, programs must focus on primary and secondary prevention, helping youth make changes in their AOD use *before* requiring more intensive treatment. Investment in prevention may lead to reduced criminal justice costs, a smaller welfare and social services burden, less need for drug and mental health treatment, and increased employment and tax revenue.

In sum, preliminary studies using MI with at-risk adolescents in a group setting are promising. Research is needed in this area to examine the short- and long-term effectiveness of group MI in reducing AOD among adolescents and to better understand how the group process may affect AOD outcomes.

ACKNOWLEDGMENTS

The D'Amico, Hunter, and Osilla study was supported by National Institute on Drug Abuse (NIDA) Grant No. R01DA019938 (Elizabeth J. D'Amico, Principal Investigator). We would also like to thank the Council in Santa Barbara and the teen court staff in Santa Barbara and Santa Maria for their support of the NIDA R01DA019938 project. The Engle, Macgowan, Wagner, and Amrhein study was made possible by three different grants from NIDA and the National Institute on Alcohol Abuse and Alcoholism (NIAAA): NIDA (No. R01 AA10246; Eric F. Wagner, Principal Investigator), NIAAA (No. 1R21AA015679-01; Mark J. Macgowan, Principal Investigator), and NIDA (No. F31 DA 020233-01A1; Brett Engle, Principal Investigator). The Bryan, Feldstein Ewing, and colleagues' study was supported by NIAAA Grant No. 1R01 AA013844-01 (Angela Bryan, Principal Investigator).

CHAPTER 19

✳ ✳ ✳ ✳

Applications in Schools

Sebastian Kaplan, Brett Engle, Ashley Austin,
and Eric F. Wagner

SCOPE OF THE PROBLEM

Adolescents experience multiple, interrelated problems that affect school performance and predict dropout, including substance abuse, peer conflict, and familial problems (Hickman, Bartholomew, & Mathwig, 2008). Recently, a growing literature base has advocated for enhanced school-based services for youth (Weist, Evans, & Lever, 2003). Wagner and Macgowan (2006) suggest that treating youth in their natural environment allows unique opportunities to directly influence proximal determinants and consequences of problem behaviors. Also, adolescents are as much as 21 times more likely to attend school-based mental health treatment than community-based care (Juszczak, Melinkovich, & Kaplan, 2003), which is critical since few adolescents who need treatment receive it (Clark, Horton, Dennis, & Babor, 2002; Dennis, Dawud-Noursi, Muck, & McDermeit, 2003).

WHY MI?

Many current school-based responses to student challenges lack empirical support, such as grade retention, "zero tolerance" policies, and Drug Abuse Resistance Education (DARE) (Adelman & Taylor, 2003; American Psychological Association Zero Tolerance Task Force, 2008; Stearns, Moller, Blau, & Potochnick, 2007). Although well-intentioned, these approaches seem to stigmatize and isolate many of the adolescents in greatest need of intervention (Dodge, Dishion, & Lansford, 2006). Furthermore, "zero tolerance" policies, which ignore contextual variables in problem behavior, create a sense of inequity or lack of fairness and reinforce beliefs about not feeling accepted in the school setting (Skiba & Peterson, 1999).

Alternatively, research supporting theory-driven and strengths-based approaches to adolescent behavior change is mounting (Nation et al., 2003). Specifically, over the last two decades, the evidence base supporting the application of MI to a variety of problems across populations has grown tremendously (Rollnick, Miller, & Butler, 2008). Many characteristics of MI are well suited to intervening with adolescents in schools.

MI SPIRIT AND STRATEGIES

MI consists of two active components: (1) A relational component involving the use of empathy and the interpersonal spirit of MI and (2) a technical component consisting of specific skills for eliciting and strengthening change talk (Miller & Rose, 2009).

MI IN SCHOOL SETTINGS

Rollnick, Miller, and Butler (2008) describe three aspects of the MI spirit: collaboration, supporting autonomy, and evocation. Collaboration relies heavily on the use of reflective listening to create a sense of acceptance. A particular challenge when working in schools is that students may perceive all adults as representatives of the school and may doubt the expressed empathy of the practitioners. Therefore, it is especially important to avoid passing judgment, offering advice without permission, or expressing criticism. For instance, if a student is frustrated with repeated office referrals, offer a reflection such as "these referrals are really getting to you." This response empathizes with the student's experience but does not condone or reinforce negative behaviors.

Supporting autonomy often begins with a mindset that accepts resistance to change as a normal human experience and involves a set of skills that enable practitioners to effectively respond in a nonconfrontational manner. The use of reflections can be especially helpful when students exhibit ambivalence toward change. For example, an empathic statement such as "You don't understand why you have been singled out to come talk to a therapist" communicates understanding and validates the student's view.

Supporting autonomy also emphasizes the student's capability and personal responsibility for change. Instead of telling the students what they "must do," students are encouraged to decide for themselves what to change. One option is to offer a menu of options rather than a mandate for change. For instance, in a conversation with a student concerned about a failing grade, identify multiple options for change and allow the student to choose what "fits" best (e.g., not smoke marijuana on school nights; get tutoring; ask teacher for help). Note such ideas and guide the student to come up with solutions herself. After the session, reflect back on the skills you used to elicit the *student's* idea. Such mental exercises are a good way to strengthen your MI skills.

Another option is to use problem solving to play out different scenarios with the student, so that he can identify the benefits and consequences of different courses of action. "You mentioned that if you only smoked marijuana on weekends, you would concentrate better." Exploring past success can help students recognize abilities that will help when facing challenges. "That would be a pretty big reduction. Have you gone the whole week without smoking in the past?" It is important to try to anticipate the student's response. If you are doubtful that the student has gone this long without using, you may ask a different question. "On a scale of 1 to 10, how confident are you that you can reduce your use?" Follow up with "Why are you not lower on the scale?" in order to elicit ability change talk.

Evoking students' thoughts, feelings, and beliefs about a problem behavior and its consequences can bring about dissonance between the behavior and students' expressed goals or values. Students can explore their current challenges (e.g., failing grades, suspensions) in relation to their professed future goals (e.g., college, make a lot of money). Cultivating student ideas about how their behavior may be contradictory to their values can be a refreshing change for students accustomed to being pressured to meet goals typically set forth by parents or teachers.

Evoking strengths is particularly important as they often contrast with problem behaviors. Highlighting strengths embedded within student statements is an advanced skill that requires practice. Among other perhaps seemingly contradictory statements, a student may communicate an important value, a reflection such as "Your health (family or career) is part of what defines you as a person." Then, give the student time and space to draw logical conclusions, which take into consideration the target behavior and the reflected value. In some cases, after establishing rapport, you may explicitly highlight the apparent contradiction. "We've talked about how you've been smoking quite a bit over the last few months. You've also said that being in great shape is critical to your performance. I wonder how these two things fit together for you."

MI AND SCHOOL PROBLEMS

The relational component of MI seeks to build a strong therapeutic alliance from which the use of technical skills can selectively elicit and reinforce a student's own arguments for change. Consider the following scenario between a student and teacher/practitioner, who have discussed the student's academic problems and substance use previously. Notice the use of targeted statements seeking to increase change talk and strengthen commitment to change.

PRACTITIONER: Alex, do you have a minute? I heard that you are failing English and I'm wondering if we could talk about it. (Asking Permission to Discuss an Identified Target Problem)

STUDENT: I'm sorry but Ms. R is just a witch. She gets on my back for no reason. Yesterday she sent me to the office. Now I have another two days in ISS [in-school suspension]. I'm telling you she's out to get me.

PRACTITIONER: You feel she treats you unfairly. (Simple Reflection; Relational Component)

STUDENT: Absolutely. She didn't say anything to the other kids. Not only do I have to deal with ISS now, I also have three tests coming up. It's getting to be too much.

PRACTITIONER: The pressure from school can really get to you at times. (Simple Reflection; Relational Component)

STUDENT: Yeah, I mean I've got enough stress.

PRACTITIONER: You've told me before that this is when you just want to escape from it all. Yet it seems you are trying to keep it together. (Reflection Leaning toward Change Talk, Reinforcing Desire to Not Use)

STUDENT: Yeah, to be honest, I was just talking with one of my friends about getting some weed this weekend. I know I said I would quit during basketball season, but (*shrugging*) . . . (Sustain Talk—Commitment Language)

PRACTITIONER: The team means a lot to you. (Complex Reflection, Selectively Reinforcing Reason to Not Use)

STUDENT: Not just playing, but my teammates and coaches are counting on me. (Change Talk—Reason to Not Use)

PRACTITIONER: You are loyal to those that rely on you (Affirmation) You are also wrestling with how you can deal with the stress from this latest incident and stay true to your decision to have the best season possible. (Complex Reflection/Summary Emphasizing Student Reasons for Not Using)

STUDENT: I guess so. I'm not saying what Ms. R did was right, but I do know if I decide to smoke weed then that could make things worse. (Change Talk—Reason to Not Use)

PRACTITIONER: You are starting to think you shouldn't get high this weekend. (Reflection Seeking Commitment Language)

STUDENT: Yeah, I'm just going to stay away from that party. I can't be smoking weed. That will just cause me more stress.

Another exercise is to develop a change plan, which occurs once the student expresses strong enough commitment to a targeted behavior change. The student works to identify (1) the steps to take to make a change. (2) people who may support her, (3) how she will know if she is being successful, and (4) potential barriers to change. The following is an example of a session with a student about "graduating on time."

STUDENT: The more I think about it, the more I realize I'm only hurting myself. I like to think that I'm having a good time but all the skipping class and partying I'm doing is only keeping me from being able to graduate on time.

PRACTITIONER: Graduating on time is your top priority. (Complex Reflection)

STUDENT: It is, and I guess it always has been, it's just that I thought all that other crap was more fun. When I think about it, there's nothing exciting about being a senior again next year.

PRACTITIONER: You're really defining what's important in your life, and right now it's getting your diploma. (Reflection of Personal Goals/Values) What is the main thing you need to focus on right now to move closer to your goals? (Looking Forward; Making a Change Plan)

STUDENT: Well, first I need to start going to class again. I know I'm going to have to deal with stupid comments from people about where I've been but whatever, I can deal. (Change Talk—Ability)

PRACTITIONER: One barrier is people criticizing you. What else might get in the way? (Open-Ended Question—Obstacles to Success)

STUDENT: All the homework I need to catch up on. It's not going to be easy to do all that. (Sustain Talk—Ability; Change Talk—Commitment)

PRACTITIONER: You stick to things when you set your mind to them no matter what. (Complex Reflection Emphasizing Commitment)

STUDENT: Yeah, I guess so. I probably need to see my teachers and find out what I need to do to catch up. (Taking Steps)

PRACTITIONER: I'm hearing that you are ready to make some changes in your classes. (Reflecting Taking Steps) Who might be able to help you do this? (Open-Ended Question—Support)

STUDENT: Definitely Mr. S, my art teacher, he's always believed in me no matter how bad I got. (Change Talk—Ability)

PRACTITIONER: People have faith in you, even some of your teachers. (Complex Reflection—Supporting Ability) So how will you know if you are on the right track? (Open-Ended Question about Tracking Success)

STUDENT: Since I'm going to start meeting with my teachers I can check in with them about my assignments. (Taking Steps) We also get progress reports in 3 weeks so I'll know more then.

In both of the above scenarios, the practitioner relies mostly on reflections, affirmations, and open-ended questions. Generally, these techniques are the foundation of MI, through which the spirit of MI, as well as the eliciting of change talk and commitment language leads to enhanced student motivation.

RESEARCH IMPLICATIONS

About a dozen mostly small scale studies have been published on the use of MI in schools. As in the broader MI literature, the application of MI in schools has been diverse, with programs targeting substance abuse (Wagner & Austin, 2009), tobacco use (Kelly & Lapworth, 2006; Woodruff, Edwards, Conway, & Elliott, 2001), as well as school conduct and academic performance (Atkinson & Woods, 2003).

McCambridge and colleagues conducted a series of larger scale studies in further education colleges for 16- to 20-year-olds in England. Combined, these studies provided mixed support for the efficacy of MI. MI's initial substance use effects diminished at the 12-month follow-up (McCambridge & Strang, 2004; 2005). Although MI did not differ from an advice condition (McCambridge, Slym, & Strang, 2008), MI did outperform an assessment-only condition for alcohol use up to 3 months (Gray, McCambridge, & Strang, 2005).

Winters and Leitten (2007) compared two brief alcohol and other drug interventions in a school setting (adolescent only; adolescent plus parent), along with a delayed treatment group control condition. Students in both MI-based treatment conditions displayed improved substance use outcomes, particularly those who received the parent component.

Other interventions have utilized MI to increase treatment engagement in school-based programs. The Motivation–Adaptive Skills–Trauma Resolution (MASTR) is a school-based protocol for conduct and academic performance problems (Greenwald, 2002). By pairing MI with other techniques, the MASTR program resulted in increased student engagement, improved family functioning, and improved behavioral and academic performance (Greenwald, 2002).

Two novel approaches to the school dropout problem have recently emerged. Rutschman and colleagues at Northeastern Illinois University developed an MI-based alternative to in-school suspension, for which preliminary analyses show as much as a 10% reduction in the dropout rate for students who received the intervention (R. Rutschman, personal communication, December 4, 2008). In addition, Daly (2006) described an effort to train recent university graduates to deliver an MI-informed intervention designed to enhance motivation to complete high school and continue toward higher education opportunities. Daly reported positive satisfaction from both the "Graduate Advocates" and the teens involved in the program ($N = 13$), all of whom graduated and continued to pursue postsecondary school training. These programs may be promising alternatives to punitive approaches traditionally used to address nonconforming behavior in high schools.

The versatility of MI allows for effectively intervening with students at a variety of different levels. A burgeoning literature supports MI-based interventions, and the school setting is widely recognized as a pivotal environment to intervene. With adequate training, mental health professionals as well as school personnel could use MI to enhance relationships with students, more effectively broach difficult topics, encourage healthy decision making, and ameliorate serious and protracted problems faced by students and schools.

✳ ✳ ✳ ✳

Family-Based Intervention

Sue Channon and Sune Rubak

SCOPE OF THE PROBLEM

A small but growing body of published work indicates the potential of MI in family-based interventions (Carroll, Libby, Sheehan, & Hyland, 2001; Channon et al., 2007; Dishion et al., 2008; Erickson, Gerstle, & Feldstein, 2005; Gance-Cleveland, 2005; Hall, Smith, & Williams, 2008; Lunkenheimer et al., 2008; Perrin, Finkle, & Benjamin, 2007; Resnicow, Davis, & Rollnick, 2006; Sindelar et al., 2004; Smith & Hall, 2007; Smith, Hall, Williams, An, & Gotman, 2006; Winickoff, Hillis, Palfrey, Perrin, & Rigotti, 2003). To maximize the possibility of engagement in family interventions, you need to be sensitive to the developmental context of the family, including family members' responses to the demands of the family life cycle, as well as the actual presentation of the distress or behaviors for which they present. Taking these developmental factors into account you also need to consider whom to see, whom to talk to, whom to hear from, in which order this is done, whether or not the consultation should include only one part of the family or all together, and vitally how to ensure the participation of all the family members in the process both within and outside of the sessions (Nock & Ferriter, 2005; Nock & Kazdin, 2005).

While Part I of this text focuses on individual work with young people, in this chapter we describe MI in the context of family-based interventions either with adolescents or younger children. To avoid overcomplication of terminology, "children" will be used for both children and young people, and "families" will be used to describe parents, other caregivers, and families with dependent children.

WHY MI?

There are challenges in translating a method developed for communication between two people (practitioner and patient) into a systemic model fit for child and family work, with all its inherent complexities. Family therapy is based on the assumption that the individual behavior needs to be understood within a family context, and it uses the family processes to create systemic change. In contrast, individual therapy traditionally focuses on individual needs, incorporating the individual's perspective on interpersonal factors.

   One of the significant differences between approaches will be whether the focus is on individual or family change. With collaboration at the heart of MI, we can respect several individuals' positions and be responsive to those different needs. MI reflects the process of good parenting, with a guiding style balanced with appropriate directing and following, representing a goodness of fit between the method and the family.

MI SPIRIT AND STRATEGIES

In the vast majority of work with children, the family is the key to the process of change. We next offer a guide for deciding when to implement family-based interventions and methods for addressing potential barriers to helping families engage in the change process.

What Should You Consider When Deciding to Implement a Family or an Individual Session?

In any presenting issue, there is a broad continuum on the level of family involvement from those where the concern is clearly something that all family members might need to address (e.g., conflict between family members) to those where it may appear quite individual (e.g., needle phobia). However, all behaviors occur in context and will impact on the evolution of family relationships. Therefore, when we are using MI with families, both family and individual counseling sessions have their place, and the MI approach will vary depending on this continuum of family involvement.

A "Whole-Family" Issue

When a family presents with a problem that they locate in the child and the parents are ambivalent in their thinking about their relationship to the problem, it can be tempting to fall into the trap of either blaming the parents or prematurely focusing on the child. This increases the risk of joining with the parents without raising the parent's related problem, and at the same time distancing the child. We need to sensitively reflect this ambivalence, explore how the parents' current actions fit with their core values as parents, while affirming their concern as parents and their wish to facilitate change for their child. In family therapy terms, this would correspond to the position of "neutrality" (Selvini, Boscolo, Cecchin, & Prata, 1980), facilitating an open-minded approach to the problem.

For example, in pediatric obesity when other family members are also obese, it is not unusual for the family to seek help for the child's weight but not reference their own weight as a related problem. The parents are often ready to help their child but not ready to look at their own ambivalence about change and its impact on the behavior. This type of situation is well suited to using MI, as ambivalence is central to the presenting problem.

When the Problem Needs Family-Based Solutions

The process of change will often require the engagement of other family members, sometimes because of the child's age, disability, or interactive nature of behavior. For example, we faced this situation in the case of an 8-year-old child with epilepsy referred because she was not going to school. She had been seizure free for a long time, and both the child and mother seemed keen for her to go to school. However, her school record of attendance was very patchy, which we understood as a reflection of both the child and parents' shared ambivalence about regular participation at school. When families present with a shared perception of ambivalence, it can be helpful to complete a shared pros and cons list, with each family member taking turns to put an item on the list. This process allows you to elicit different statements for understanding their different issues, while allowing the conversation to remain a joint and family-focused exercise. Once a list has been generated, it is important to establish for each family member what is most important to them, what they feel they can change, and to help develop a change plan. Also, it is sometimes helpful to prioritize the child's choice on which factor to handle first (in this case it was setting up a school meeting). This shows the children that they are the center of obtaining behavioral change and that the family will provide the actual support needed to help them follow through with the new behavior.

When the Difficulties Occur Mostly at Home and Not in the School Environment

For most parents, the child's display of behavioral issues predominantly in the home can have a significant impact on their own parental self-efficacy. For example, parents can perceive the child's behavior as a result of their own parenting practices, or even that the child is doing it "deliberately" to spite them. In exploring these issues, it may be appropriate to use positive reframing skills, such as guiding the parent to discuss situations where the child demonstrates more prosocial behaviors and the parent similarly can display effective positive parenting skills. With permission, parents may also benefit from advice about the normative aspects of children's misbehavior as occurring in contexts where they feel safest, such as the home.

Even when parents are offered normative feedback, we have found that many remain ambivalent about treatment recommendations, and often they lack sufficient information about the child's actual behavior. Therefore, by raising awareness and responding to parental concerns with the core MI skills, such as empathy and use of reflections, the use of brief advice can serve to decrease their ambivalence. In this way, parents can be helped to place less blame on self and others for the behavior, and be more able to be supportive to the child's level of need and actual behavior change goals (Hall et al., 2008; Smith et al., 2006; Smith & Hall, 2007).

When Changes Will Affect the Entire Family Unit

Families are constantly evolving, and every behavior change impacts on family members to some degree. As some changes (or lack thereof) can be more significant, one useful way to conceptualize and frame the change process on the family is in terms of family life-cycle themes. For example, if a 12-year-old with diabetes learns to handle his own injections, it is an age-appropriate, positive step to his becoming more independent. However, as children's autonomous behaviors begin to increase, parents will need to adjust their parenting practices to match the child's emerging needs for independence. Thus, by understanding the family's developmental transitions and cycles, you can foster the process of change.

When Is It Preferable Not to See the Family?

There are situations when directing your intervention individually to either the parents and/or children is the preferred course of treatment. Similarly, at other times, starting with a family focus and then transitioning to an individually based focus can be more appropriate. We next review four key questions you might consider when tailoring your intervention to the family.

Does the Family Display High Levels of Conflict?

When the child and parent present with diametrically opposing views, it can prove very difficult to prevent sessions from becoming a reenactment of the conflicts at home. If you find that you have difficulties engaging family members, consider individually based sessions, and revisit options for family-based intervention at a later time.

If you choose to proceed with a family-focused intervention, it is important to remain neutral and facilitate while not taking sides. Conflicts are often expressions of ambivalence in the family concerning the behavior. Therefore it is important to focus on the impact of the conflict on relationships throughout the family, and not be tempted to try to solve the conflict. Maintaining a focus on historical family times that were positive for the entire family can also serve to help the family reflect on the history of the conflict (and provides information about the relationship) rather than thinking about how to solve (or continue with) the current conflict.

Are the Family Members at Very Different Stages of the Change Process?

Family members can often be at dissimilar stages in their goals for change. For example, this is common when an older teenager is more ready to think about change than her parents and is in a position to make the changes independently. Similarly, parents may be willing to make large-scale changes, while the child is not yet ready to take on multiple behavioral goals for change.

Does the Family Hold Powerful Beliefs for How You Should Intervene?

Some families come with a very clear belief that the work should be done mostly with the child. With these families, solutions are viewed as stemming from the child, and parents see their role as minimal in the change process. By remaining MI consistent and offering the family options that best suit them, you can prevent family dropout and keep options open to possibly initiate a family focus if and when the family becomes more agreeable to this type of intervention.

Are the Presenting Issues an Adult Area for Intervention Rather Than Family?

Deciphering family versus adult parental treatment issues can sometimes be difficult, particularly when you are just beginning to work with a family. In general, we find that when treatment issues present in which the child has no volitional control, such as domestic violence or parental substance abuse, family-based interventions should be avoided and individual treatment initiated first.

RESEARCH IMPLICATIONS

Given the limited research in family-based MI interventions, there is a need for long-term evaluation of MI's effectiveness in relation to work with children and families in these contexts. We need to understand how to achieve the best fit between MI and family-focused work and how to generalize from research to everyday practice. Certainly, MI can offer much to family interventions, and we believe the next research challenge of the field is to identify the key components of MI that can help to facilitate behavioral changes that will match both the developmental and contextual needs of families.

PART III

* * *

CHOOSING YOUR OWN PATH

CHAPTER 21

❋　　❋　　❋　　❋

Ethical Considerations

> The more sophisticated your ethics get, the stronger you have
> to be to stay afloat. And when you say good-bye to objective
> values, you really have to flex your muscles and keep your eyes
> open, because you are on your own.
> —JOHN BARTH, *The End of the Road*

A general review of ethics has been described in previous MI texts (see Miller & Rollnick, 2002; Rollnick, Miller, & Butler, 2008), and we encourage you to review these chapters. Our focus in this part of the book involves how these general ethical principles in MI can be extended and incorporated in your work with young persons and families.

INFLUENCE, VALUES, AND GOALS

Influence: Is It Always Present?

Although MI principles encapsulate the ethical principles of respect, benevolence, and autonomy, we believe the issue of influence is always present in any behavior change intervention. Your role as a guide by definition involves exerting influence on another person no matter how collaborative the goal may be. When the person's values and goals are associated with what you believe to be positive change, your influence is consistent with what the person already wants. However, when you believe the person's values or goals do not maximize his or her potential or are in fact harmful, you may experience what Miller and Rollnick (2002) coin "ethical itches." These are the nagging concerns you may feel when guiding the person toward goals you consider healthy but inconsistent with the person's choices. In MI with young people and families, your influence in the change process can become even trickier than in work with adults, in that you are balancing the goals of the young person, other family members, and sometimes multiple treatment providers. Each may have his or her own agenda for behavior change, and figuring out what and whose goals you are targeting can be a feat in and of itself!

As Miller and Rollnick (2002) note, there is nothing wrong with these itches, and it is a tribute to your own ethics that you can feel the itch. To help soothe you, we next offer a guide, based on the ethical guidelines of Miller and Rollnick, to help you maintain your focus on maximizing the young person's potential and not falling into a trap of your own or of others' biases and values. The first step is to clarify each player's values and goals in order to pave the way for open and honest communication about behavior change.

Values and Goals of the Young Person:
Is This Always Most Important?

Ideally, your use of MI with young people targets their behavior change goals. The young person would present with a goal in mind, request your help, and the change process would roll. Often however, as we note throughout the text, the young person's aspirations for change aren't always clear. Sometimes, they are even counter to what you can offer. For example, a common frustration reported by pediatricians and child psychiatrists occurs when young people come in asking or demanding certain medical services the physician does not deem to be medically indicated: the college student who wants a stimulant to help him stay awake to study, or the high school student who heard that benzodiazepines would help her be less anxious during exam time. When these occasions occur, it is appropriate to ask the young person not only what he or she wants, but as Miller and Rollnick (2002) suggest, "What do you want from me?"

Values and Goals of the Family: How Much Do They Matter?

It is important to consider the values and goals of the family that is seeking your help, not only because you bear an obligation to the legal guardians of the young person but also because family members' values and goals can both help and hinder the young person's changes. For example, consider a young female wanting to lose weight. She identifies the nightly family meal as her biggest obstacle to reducing caloric intake, although the mealtime is the family's valued tradition. Your consideration to invite the young person's parent(s) into this discussion (with her permission) can powerfully affect how changes in her behavior could take place, as well as impact how the family is (or is not) willing to support her changes. As a general rule, how you encourage family members to voice their concerns and goals for young people can clearly enhance what and how change is supported in the natural environment outside of your clinic office.

At the same time, family goals for the young person can sometimes offer challenges. Family members can often present with a treatment agenda that differs from what the practitioner wants or has to offer. In the case of a young person seeking stimulants to help him study, the family members may have differing ideas, may be supportive of this goal, not know of the young person's wishes, or be against this decision. Again, we believe it is important to frankly discuss with family members, as well as the young person, not only what they want from treatment, but also what they want from you as the MI practitioner.

Values and Goals of the Practitioner: Does What You Want Matter?

Miller and Rollnick (2002) discuss three types of values practitioners may have in doing MI: compassion, opinion, and investment. *Compassion* refers to a selfless and caring concern for the other person's welfare and his or her best interest. For example, a mother demonstrates compassion when she listens without offering advice while her daughter cries on her shoulder after her first relationship breakup. With young people, your compassion may evolve into a strong caregiver instinct to protect the young person from engaging in risk. You must take extra care to ensure that this instinct does not cloud your respect for autonomy and personal choice.

Opinion involves a professional judgment as to which decision serves the young person's best interest. Young people may ask for a professional opinion, and family members and other treatment providers will often do so. In rendering an opinion, Miller and Rollnick (2002), suggest you consider what the outcomes would be for the young person in resolving their own ambivalence in one direction or the other if an opinion is given. Would this help or hinder, and how will you know? When working with young people, you must take extra care to identify generational or cultural gaps in terms of what you believe are appropriate behaviors, responsibilities, and environments for a young person versus what may be normative in their contexts.

Investment describes a personal gain or loss to you, depending on the young person's ultimate decision. Investments can take several forms. For example, a practitioner working in a private, for-profit agency may have a material investment in the young person enrolling in treatment. A practitioner who has experienced similar life issues as the young person or family member, such as substance abuse, may have a symbolic investment in the young person engaging in change. Again, we do not provide a foolproof ointment for these itches. Rather, we believe that your awareness and thoughtful balancing of these concerns will result in the best outcome for the young person.

Values and Goals of Other Treatment Providers: How Do They Play a Role?

Young people spend their lives in multiple contexts (i.e., school, relationships with peers and family, work, religious settings, and with other treatment providers, etc.) where other adults have their own agendas for the young person's goals and values. You may find it challenging to coordinate your work with other treatment providers, especially those providers who are taking a more directive approach (e.g., legal system) or those who instill a sense of urgency due to the life-threatening nature of the young person's behavior (e.g., health care system). Common examples include young people struggling with substance abuse who are told by the treatment provider they must remain abstinent from all alcohol and drugs, but the parents expect only moderation in use, or the young person who is medically fragile and may be considering a break from the treatment regimen, although these changes are not supported by their medical practitioner or family. In these situations, we again believe the best interest of the young person is served by asking other practitioners not only their treatment aspirations, but also what they would like from you as a collaborator in helping the young person to change. It may also be helpful to elicit from providers how directive approaches and/or threatening stances have not worked with the young person thus far (see Chapter 3, elicit–provide–elicit). In these situations, your use of OARS (see Chapter 4) can demonstrate empathy for the other providers' point of view and assure them that you hear their concerns.

Managing Multiple Agendas: How Is It Possible?

As you can see, values and goals are not always congruent in your work with young persons and families. In the times when all partners are dancing to the same tune and goals for change are in agreement, you are well on your way to behavioral activation. In contrast, when agendas differ and each of the dancing partners wants to do a different dance, questions of how to set goals for change often arise.

Examples

A young girl struggling academically wants her pediatrician to prescribe her a stimulant to help her focus because she thinks she has attention problems. The pediatrician does not believe she has a diagnosis to justify the use of medication, while the girl's counselor is in support of this diagnosis and originally recommended the consult for services. The parent is against the girl taking medication, but does not want to create conflict in the relationship with her daughter, and will support whatever decision is made.

A young adult male convicted of driving while under the influence is referred for court-mandated counseling and is advised by the judge to remain abstinent from alcohol. The counselor would like to pursue a goal of controlled drinking. The young man is not interested in selecting a goal, does not want to stop drinking, and only wants to attend counseling to complete his probation.

The values and goals of young persons and other adults often diverge. When these divergent perspectives are still ultimately about maximizing the young person's potential, MI is ethically appropriate as long as you are honest about the behavior change goal. Miller and Rollnick (2002) posit that the ethical principle of benevolence prevails during these occasions, as the other person holds objective value and judgment in what is in the young person's best interest. We agree that the issue of benevolence holds merit under these circumstances, particularly when the young person is engaging in risk behaviors (i.e., substance abuse or not complying with medically necessary treatments), and when he or she lacks the insight to stay free from harm. Of course, if the young person is truly at risk of immediate harm, MI is not appropriate, and you may need to violate autonomy to keep the patient safe.

You should use MI with caution when others have a personal investment in the young person changing beyond maximizing the young person's potential. Examples include a parent who wants the young person to be the first in the family to attend college when the young person seeks to obtain vocational skills. Another example of personal investment beyond maximizing potential is the young person who seeks to learn controlled drinking skills but whose parents or medical provider wants to set a goal of abstinence owing to their own history of alcohol misuse. You may still want to engage the young person in MI sessions during these situations, but you will need to be very clear to other adults that the goals you set will be collaborative with the young person.

Finally, if you as the practitioner are in a position of power and the young person can experience consequences as the result of what they tell you, MI is not appropriate. For example, if you are a probation officer interviewing a young person suspected of selling marijuana and the information you obtain could lead to further involvement with the law, you should not use MI.

GUIDELINES FOR ETHICAL PRACTICE: DOING THE RIGHT THING

We have discussed what not to do when using MI with young persons and families, and next conclude with some helpful examples and guidelines initially proposed by Miller and Rollnick (2002). In considering how you can balance ethics and MI, we suggest you continue to follow the ethical standards of your profession as well. Furthermore, when you feel an ethical itch, don't ignore or avoid it: Scratch it some, but make it go away and heal. Do something about it, and don't let it fester. As in the journey of learning MI, dealing with ethical issues is a process. Once you think you know how to play the game, a curve ball can get thrown at you. What we hope is that you will be able to be flexible when these occasions arise and use these additional guidelines as a resource to facilitate a more productive encounter focused on the young person's engagement in change.

Guideline 1: When you perceive disagreement in the therapeutic relationship or an area of ethical malaise, clarify everyone's agenda (including your own).

Example 1

A counselor working with a young male was referred for substance abuse treatment by the legal system. The judge has mandated 20 visits and requires weekly urinalysis testing (other's aspiration). When the youth comes to the clinic, he states he does not want to talk about his marijuana use, but instead wants the counselor's help in learning to be less anxious around new people (young person's aspiration). The counselor only focuses on the youth's substance misuse, decides that because he is court-mandated and it is what the judge aspires for treatment, this is the only viable option. The counselor proceeds to use MI only on topics he deems pertinent to substance misuse.

OUR OPINION: UNETHICAL USE OF MI

While the young person is referred for substance abuse treatment, the counselor does not clarify with the young person how his goals for treatment may or may not be in accord with the goals of the judge or counselor, and disregards his aspirations. A more ethical approach to using MI would have been to clarify the discrepancy between the aspirations of the young person, judge, and counselor, explore how the young person's aspirations for change might be related to his substance misuse, and then set an agenda for the focus of treatment.

Guideline 2: When your opinion as to what is in the young person's best interest is in disagreement with what the young person wants, reevaluate and collaborate about your agenda, making known your own concerns and goals for the young person.

Example 2

A pediatrician is asked by a young teen to prescribe a stimulant (young person's aspiration). Although she has not been formally evaluated, the girl believes she has attention problems, and her counselor agrees she needs medication (other's aspiration). The mother of the girl is ambivalent and will agree to whatever decision is made (other's aspiration). As a diagnosis has not been made, the pediatrician is not willing to ethically prescribe medication without proper evaluation (other's aspiration). The pediatrician listens to the young person and others' aspirations, and then asks permission to discuss them collaboratively. With permission from the youth, she explains to her the ethical concerns about prescribing at this time, and together, the young person and pediatrician set up a plan for her to complete an evaluation and return for follow-up with the results. The next course of treatment will be discussed at that time. The young person, counselor, pediatrician, and mother all end in agreement.

OUR OPINION: ETHICAL USE OF MI

The pediatrician incorporated the spirit of MI, asked permission to discuss her concerns, and explored each person's aspirations. A collaborative agenda was set, and options for follow-up were provided. Each person's aspirations were validated, while the pediatrician maintained an ethical stance in providing appropriate care.

Guideline 3: *The greater your personal investment in the young person's outcome, the more unacceptable it is to use MI. When your personal investment is not in accord with the young person's best interests, MI is inappropriate.*

Example 3

A medical resident working on an inpatient unit is working with his first patient hospitalized for juvenile diabetes. The young male is 75 pounds overweight, does not maintain proper glucose levels, and is hospitalized at least monthly for his poor self-care regimen. The resident suspects that if the youth continues to neglect his health, he may meet death by the age of 21. Each day, the resident thinks about ways to help the young male, and checks on him regularly during the day, even though the youth is not on his service. The resident has recently learned MI and decides to try to use it with the young man to help him become more compliant with his health regimen. He structures the consultation to include specific strategies, such as the looking forward and rulers' exercises. However, when the young man tells him he isn't ready to talk about the future—it's just too far away—the resident becomes upset and tells the young man he is going to die if he doesn't change.

OUR OPINION: UNETHICAL USE OF MI

The medical resident in this example is more invested than the youth in altering his health habits, and the manner in which MI was used in this case is unacceptable. Rather than offering the young man opportunities to voice his own goals and values about health, the resident is the one doing all of the work and, in effect, elicits only sustain talk. Moreover, the resident overextends his professional obligations, visiting with the young man when he is not on his service, and spends his own free time considering options he deems are best for the youth. A more ethical approach to using MI in this example would have been for the resident first to consult with the young man only when he was on his service. Second, the resident should have used the MI spirit and allowed the young man to select his own valued topics and goals to discuss. Last, by displaying a neutral stance in the young person's decision to discuss health behavior change options, the resident would have enhanced the youth's autonomy and created a more open path for him to explore his motivation to change.

Guideline 4: When your role involves coercive power to influence the young person's behavior and outcomes, a higher degree of caution is warranted. If coercive power is combined with personal investment in the young person's behavior and outcomes, MI is inappropriate.

Example 4

After being arrested for selling marijuana, a 16-year-old male was brought to his first visit with his probation officer by his adoptive mother. The probation officer recently underwent an agencywide training in MI and decides to incorporate it into her assessment. She immediately begins her interaction with the youth by conveying the spirit of MI while balancing her goals of assessment. During the interview, she often mentions to the young person that she "likes to keep my caseload light," and expects that he "will do everything as he is told to get off probation as quickly as possible." She "really doesn't like to send kids to juvenile detention." As the interview continues, the youth becomes less communicative and the probation officer attends to this feedback, realizing she has not been truly using MI. With this realization, she returns to using MI and again notices a shift in the young person's response to her. She proceeds to set a collaborative agenda, asks permission multiple times throughout the rest of interview, continues to convey the spirit of MI, and also includes the mother's aspirations for her son into the probation goals. At the end of the interview, specific goals are set, with the probation officer, youth, and parent stating agreement to the plan.

OUR OPINION: ETHICAL USE OF MI

The probation officer in this scenario is placed in a difficult situation. She has to set clear limitations with the young person and holds a high level of coercive power. Throughout the majority of the interaction, the probation officer effectively incorporated MI and met the goals of the visit. While she did briefly broach the unethical, by touting her power and reminding the young person that she has authority to place him in juvenile detention if he is noncompliant with his probation plan, she was able to respond accordingly to the young person when he began to disengage, and she did not breach ethics. Situations that place providers in such power-yielding roles often increase the likelihood of venturing off the MI path. However, by staying present and responding to the best teacher of MI, the young person, returning to the path can efficiently result in remaining ethical when using MI.

In summary, we hope we have provided a foundation for you to recognize ethical itches. Your first job is to clarify and understand the agendas of all parties (youth, family, other providers, and yourself). The next steps are variable, depending on the unique situations and your use of MI. You may find it helpful to discuss any ethical issues with your supervisor or peers to assist in clarifying your own agenda as well as a course of action. What do you think you will do the next time you experience an ethical itch?

CHAPTER 22

✳ ✳ ✳ ✳

Developing Proficiency
in Motivational Interviewing

> You must *be* the change you want to see in the world.
> —MAHATMA GHANDI

As with any change process, incorporating MI into your clinical repertoire involves thoughtful consideration and practice. We hope you will view the pyramid as a roadmap for learning and as a skill set you will continually refine over time. Similar to playing an instrument, a few lessons are not sufficient to become proficient, and even skilled musicians often seek additional training. In addition, we hope we have conveyed to you the idea that the process of change can be as hard for practitioners as it is for young people. The goals you set for yourself for learning MI will be individualized, and we hope you use this book as a guide rather than as a prescription. You may choose to focus on small goals within each level of the pyramid, attend to a single skill, tackle all the skills in the order presented, or choose the skills most relevant for you. Of course, we hope you will carry the MI spirit into all your work with young people. We next review options for further training to highlight the next steps you might take in your own journey of change.

FUTURE DIRECTIONS FOR LEARNING MI

Now that you know the steps involved in MI, how might you practice these skills and further develop your clinical repertoire? Over the last two decades, exponential growth has taken place in opportunities for learning

MI and in methods for measuring practitioner competence. Research studies on what it takes to effectively learn MI are beginning to emerge. We next review several of these learning possibilities and hope this review will provide further guidance as to how you can continue to become more adept in your use of MI with young persons and families.

What Does It Take to Learn MI?

The art of becoming a skilled MI practitioner involves a learning process, much akin to becoming proficient in any complex musical instrument or sport. Several studies have investigated what it takes to effectively learn MI. Attending at least 2 or 3 days of an MI workshop is necessary to gain a beginning level of MI proficiency, and practitioners with less training have not been able to demonstrate basic skills (Miller et al., 2008). Skill gains have been found for professionals in a variety of settings, with at least a 2- to 3-day training workshop, such as probation (Miller & Mount, 2005); mental health therapists (Schoener, Madeja, Henderson, Ondersma, & Janisse, 2006); substance abuse (Moyers et al., 2008; Tober et al., 2005); as well as medical specialties (dieticians; Brug et al., 2007), medical students (Martino, Haesler, Belitsky, Pantalon, & Fortin, 2007), residents (Chossis et al., 2007), specialist nurses (Lane, Johnson, Rollnick, Edwards, & Lyons, 2003), and general practitioners (Rubak, Sandlbaek, Lauritzen, Borch-Johnsen, & Christensen, 2006). However, we have also learned that after practitioners participated in a 2-day workshop alone, patient outcomes did not improve (e.g., change talk does not increase (Miller et al., 2004).

What matters most in your journey of learning MI is not the initial steps you take, but how you choose to proceed down the path. These steps include engaging in coaching and feedback from a person more knowledgeable in MI than you. Said in other words, if you don't use it, you lose it. For example, in a large-scale study, Miller and colleagues (2004) compared the learning of MI via self-directed methods (reading and watching videotapes) to receiving workshop training followed by one of four conditions: no additional services, coaching, written feedback on audiotaped sessions, and coaching plus written feedback. While all of the conditions evidenced an increase in MI skill acquisition post training, results in proficiency differed. Those participants in the condition that received coaching plus feedback post training displayed the greatest skill proficiency, while workshop-only participants displayed a regression in their skills toward their initial baseline skill level.

The research on training from Miller and colleagues (2004) and others demonstrates that the process of gaining proficiency in MI requires your time: time to learn, time to practice, time to receive feedback, and time in general. How much time is required? The verdict is still out. Consider if you were to walk down a path for 5 minutes versus 5 hours. Either way you make progress, but with a greater time investment you will get further along the trail. The same idea holds true when learning MI. Proficiency in MI, like most skills, is a lifelong journey.

Learning to Crawl: Self-Study

Books in Guilford's Applications of Motivational Interviewing series offer content tailored to mental health, health care, and training, and several MI videos are available (see *www.motivationalinterviewing.org*). Observing MI encounters is helpful to bring texts to life. An excellent "self-help" book is Rosengren's *Building Motivational Interviewing Skills: A Practitioner Workbook* (2009), complete with self-training quizzes and exercises for each level of the pyramid. These methods can surely increase your understanding of MI and expose you to how MI might be used with young persons. However, they will never substitute for practice. Books and videos provide a "ground school for flying" (Miller, Sorensen, Selzer, and Brigham, 2006), but you cannot get a flying license without a flying instructor. We recognize time constraints often limit practitioners from moving beyond self-study. The difficulty in becoming proficient in MI only by these passive methods is they leave you disengaged and nonactive in the learning process (i.e., reading about MI is not doing MI).

Learning to Walk: Attend a Training Workshop

When first introduced to MI, many of us are drawn to the core humanistic qualities of the style. The openness, respect for autonomy, and overall valuing of the young person's journey often resonate with our own professional values of caring for this often neglected population. Similarly, when initially learning MI, it is common to believe MI is easy to do—just listen, ask certain questions, and use the skills. However, when practitioners begin to try out MI with young persons after initially reading a text or watching videos, they often quickly gain a deeper appreciation of the level of difficulty in implementing even seemingly simple tasks (e.g., reflections). Typically, the more you grasp MI, the more you recognize what more you need to learn. If you are at this point, attendance at a 2- or 3-day training workshop often is a good next step in the learning process.

So what can you expect from a general training MI training workshop? In general, by attending an initial workshop, you will have a greater understanding of the underlying spirit and basic style of MI, recognize reflective listening responses and differentiate them from other counseling responses, increase your skills for providing reflective listening responses (up to 50%), practice other active listening skills and strategies to roll with resistance, recognize change talk and differentiate commitment language from other types of change talk, and be able to list and demonstrate differing strategies for eliciting change talk. In addition, with the increase in training workshops tailored to practitioners working with young persons, it is our hope that issues of development and family processes, as well as use of video analysis and real-time role plays designed with the issues central to the young person, will also be incorporated into these trainings.

Learning to Dance: Access Coaching and Feedback

After initially learning MI in an introductory workshop, research has shown that to achieve any significant gain in MI skills, participation in a combination of ongoing personal feedback and performance coaching is crucial (Miller et al., 2004). In other words, practice without feedback can sometimes be more detrimental to your learning MI than no practice at all. When you continue to play a piece of music incorrectly without feedback, it can be even more difficult to unlearn later.

So what can you expect from these coaching and feedback sessions? First, it is important to work with someone who is more skillful in MI than you. They will have more experience and likely also have undergone their own supervision when learning MI. Coaches also serve as learning tools, with some examples including observing role plays with other supervisees and structuring feedback from the group, teaching you to code your own and other taped MI encounters, and helping to coordinate and supervise peer-mentoring groups (both are discussed in the next session). Also important in your work with a coach is the emphasis on your receiving feedback and practicing skills for effectively monitoring and responding to the young person's developmental needs, as well the contextual familial issues that often present during an MI encounter.

In order to give you feedback, your coach will need to hear you do MI. This often involves listening to your tapes (much the way a dance teacher would need to watch you dance to know if you have learned the proper steps). Taped encounters are typically discussed, with the supervisee having a collaborative role in both listening to the visit and discussing what skills they practiced, as well as receiving feedback from the coach about their practice. Feedback is given both verbally and objectively. Often, standardized coding systems are used to assess progress and monitor the MI's fidelity.

We next briefly review two of those most commonly MI coding systems typically used with adult populations: the Motivational Interviewing Skill Code (MISC) Scale (Moyers, Martin, Catley, Harris, & Ahluwalia, 2003), and the Motivational Interviewing Treatment Integrity (MITI) Scale (Moyers et al., 2003, 2005). Both share in common the use of audio- or videotaping of sessions, and at minimum a 20-minute review of the encounter for coding. Each holds its own merit for use, depending on what type of question you are seeking to answer in your analysis of the MI encounter. The MISC 2.0 is a more intensive coding system that yields behavior counts for both practitioner and patient. The MITI is a briefer coding system that yields ratings for the practitioner only. We offer this summary, not as some-thing you should bank in memory, but rather as a resource to help you master your MI dance steps. Your use of coding systems can also facilitate your understanding of what skills you may need to refine, as well as allow for a more detailed analysis of the MI encounter that can be obtained from just listening to a tape. Finally, we note that although these validated cod-ing systems are highly effective in providing a detailed analysis of your encounter, neither was specifically designed for young persons and families, and as of yet, an MI coding system has not been validated for use with this population.

The MISC 2.0

Originally developed in 1997, the MISC offers a behavioral coding system for extensive analysis of the MI method and is often used in process research investigating the critical elements and causal mechanisms of MI. The MISC codes both the practitioner's MI consistent behaviors and patient language; thus the MISC can be used to link practitioner communication with patient outcomes. The MISC system involves three separate reviews of your taped encounter. The first is a set of global practice ratings of the practitioner's style, response of the young person, and quality of the interaction. The sec-ond analysis involves a review of your responses (e.g., open-ended question, closed question, reflection, advice, giving information) and the young per-son's utterances (e.g., change and sustain talk) using a system of mutually exclusive behavior categories. The third pass records your and the young person's talk time and documents each person's percentage of talk time.

The MITI 3.0

The MITI is the child of MISC 2.0, but assesses only practitioner behav-iors. As with any family, they share commonalities and goals in evaluating MI skills via behavioral methods, but serve different functions. While the MISC has been used for more detailed process research investigating the critical elements and causal mechanisms, the MITI provides a briefer evalu-ation of the level of MI spirit and the frequency of MI consistent behaviors. The MITI involves only a one-pass review, with two major components, the global and behavior count scores. The global scores capture the rat-er's global impression or overall judgment about two dimensions of the MI encounter: empathy/understanding and spirit. From this, each MITI review will contain two global scores, with the dimension referred to as the "gestalt." The behavior count score involves your tallying the instances of specific practitioner behaviors, which include giving information in an MI adherent or nonadherent manner, and classifying questions (open and closed) and reflections (simple and complex).

How Do I Find a Dance Instructor?

If you or your agency is interested in pursuing training, there is currently no formal certification for becoming an MI trainer. However, the international Motivational Interviewing Network of Trainers (MINT) promotes quality MI training by offering Train the Trainer workshops. We recommend seeking training from members of MINT who are actively aware of updates in MI research and training approaches. MINT operates an informational website (*www.motivationalinterview.org*) offering information about MI and providing a geographical listing of MINT members. To date, training has been provided internationally in at least 27 languages. If you are seeking a trainer with expertise in MI and young people, the MINT listing includes information about trainers' specialty areas. We recommend you ask potential trainers how much expertise they have in MI with young people and families and request references or evaluations from prior training workshops.

Learning to Dance with Others: Establish an MI Learning Group with Peers

One of the pitfalls of having a coach outside your organization is that he or she is not always available. Establishing your own MI learning group with peers provides an alternative if having a coach is not possible, yet the core goals of strengthening MI skills remain the same.

So what are the steps and goals of a peer group? Rosengren (2009) has offered the following recommendations as a guide:

Schedule Routine Meetings

Offer times that are conducive to the group members' work schedule. Rosengren advises selecting times that are frequent (i.e., bi-weekly) but not overly intrusive as to make them cumbersome to work schedules (i.e., weekly), or too minimal to maintain group goals (i.e., monthly). Also important in structuring your meetings are taking care of practical matters (e.g., coordinating tape reviews and agenda setting).

Use an Agenda, but Don't Be Rigid

Much akin to the menu of options you might offer to the young person during an encounter, the use of an agenda in your group meetings can help participants to know what will happen and the best way to learn from the group meeting. A second option involves structuring the groups to coincide with the stages of learning, such as in this text, and emphasize skills accordingly. The third option proposed by Rosengren involves the use of meetings (especially those at the initial stage), as a vehicle for learning more about MI—for example, including time to review and discuss articles relevant to MI with young persons and/or families, or the MINT Bulletin.

Practice

If there is one golden rule in learning MI, we believe it is "practice." Reviewing training exercises and practicing them in your group with peers can be particularly helpful. Discuss challenges, skills you are learning, and skills on which you next plan to focus.

Review Tapes for Expert MI Practice

Observing practitioners that do MI can be an excellent model for learning. A list of training videos can be found on the MI website.

Code Your Own and Others' Tapes

Listening and coding tapes can enhance your knowledge of MI as you listen for links between practitioner skills and client language. Coding systems can range from the simplistic (i.e., counting client change talk and practitioner response) to the more formalized (i.e., MITI). Of course, you must first ensure that the young person has agreed to be audiotaped and to have tapes reviewed for training purposes. We have found that most young persons are generally agreeable to being taped when you tell them you are interested in learning how you might be a better practitioner and you are evaluating yourself, not them. When listening to the tapes of others, remember to respond in an MI fashion by expressing empathy and supporting self-efficacy.

Consult about Challenging Situations

When you are experiencing frustration or feeling stuck, group members often have valuable and creative suggestions about how to use MI in these situations. Ideas can not only be discussed, but can also develop into helpful role plays. You may play the young person and have another practitioner demonstrate a unique approach. Then, you may follow by trying out alternative responses to the difficult interaction in a subsequent role play.

Consider Additional Targeted Training

When particular challenges arise, such that peers feel similarly stuck, or when difficulties common to the group arise in several peer sessions, it may be helpful to seek targeted training. Approaching an MI trainer with a specific request (e.g., a coaching session around negotiating change plans; how to handle chronic ambivalence) can lead to a valuable consultation that can move you and your peers forward in learning MI.

IF YOU DON'T USE IT, YOU LOSE IT

Miller and Rollnick (2002) suggest that one of the best ways to learn MI and improve your skills is to listen to the feedback and guidance you receive from the young persons and families you serve. They will be your best teachers. Remember that the process of your learning and doing MI is much akin to a young person's journey of development and change, and one that will be unique to you. What we hope you will take from this is that there is no one right way "to do" MI. It takes two to tango to MI, and when you are working with young people, it often takes three, four, or more, depending on the size of the family!

Recall also that practice over time with guided feedback is the key to becoming proficient. This mantra applies even once you are well down the path of having learned MI. If you stop playing your instrument, your skills will fade. After initially acquiring MI skills, the final and ongoing step involves the generalization and continued refinement of these skills. We have provided several suggestions for continuing your own journey of change, including workshop attendance, coaching and supervision, review of taped sessions, peer supervision, and, most importantly, listening to the talk of young people. These are all paths for you to choose in your journey of learning MI. Which one will you choose next?

References

Adelman, H. S., & Taylor, L. (2003). Creating school and community partnerships for substance abuse prevention programs. *Journal of Primary Prevention, 23*, 329–369.

Agency for Healthcare Research and Quality (AHRQ). (2008). *Treating tobacco use and dependence: 2008 update* (U.S. Public Health Service Clinical Practice Guideline Executive Summary). Washington, DC. Author.

American Psychiatric Association. (2000). *Diagnostic and statistical manual of mental disorders* (4th ed., text rev.). Washington, DC: Author.

American Psychological Association Zero Tolerance Task Force. (2008). Are zero tolerance policies effective in the schools?: An evidentiary review and recommendations. *American Psychologist, 63*, 852–862.

Amrhein, P. C., Miller, W. R., Yahne, C. E., Palmer, M., & Fulcher, L. (2003). Client commitment language during motivational interviewing predicts drug use outcomes. *Journal of Consulting and Clinical Psychology, 71*, 862–878.

Anhalt, K., & Morris, T. L. (1998). Developmental and adjustment issues of gay, lesbian, and bisexual adolescents: A review of the empirical literature. *Clinical Child and Family Psychology Review, 1*, 215–230.

Arkowitz, H. & Westra, H. A. (2004). Integrating motivational interviewing and cognitive behavioural therapy in the treatment of depression and anxiety. *Journal of Cognitive Psychotherapy, 18*, 337–350.

Arnett, J. J. (2000). Emerging adulthood: A theory of development from the late teens through the twenties. *American Psychologist, 55*, 469–480.

Arnett, J. J. (2001). Conceptions of the transition to adulthood: Perspectives from adolescence to midlife. *Journal of Adult Development 8*, 133–143.

Arnett, J. J. (2004). *Emerging adulthood: The winding road from the late teens through the twenties.* New York: Oxford University Press.

Ashman, J. J., Conviser, R., & Pounds, M. B. (2002). Associations between HIV-positive individuals' receipt of ancillary services and medical care receipt and retention, *AIDS Care, 14*, s109–118.

Atkinson, C., & Woods, K. (2003). Motivational interviewing strategies for disaffected secondary school students: A case example. *Educational Psychology in Practice, 19*, 49–64.

Backinger C. L., Fagan, P., Matthews, E., & Grana, R. A. (2003). Adolescent and young adult tobacco prevention and cessation: Current status and future directions. *Tobacco Control, 12*(Suppl. 4), IV46–53.

Baer, J. S., Beadnell, B., Garrett, S. B., Hartzler, B., Wells, E. A., & Peterson, P. L. (2008). Adolescent change language within a brief motivational intervention and substance use outcome. *Psychology of Addictive Behaviors, 22*, 570–575.

Baer, J., Stacy, A., & Larimer, M. (1991, November). Biases in the perception of drinking norms among college students. *Journal of Studies on Alcohol, 52*(6), 580–586.

Bailey, K. A., Baker, A. L., Webster, R. A., & Lewin, T. J. (2004). Pilot randomized controlled trial of a brief alcohol intervention group for adolescents. *Drug and Alcohol Review, 23*(2), 157–166.

Barrowclough, C., Haddock, G., Tarrier, N., Lewis, S. W., Moring, J., O'Brien, R., et al. (2001). Randomized controlled trial of motivational interviewing, cognitive behavior therapy, and family intervention for patients with comorbid schizophrenia and substance use disorders. *American Journal of Psychiatry, 158*, 1706–1713.

Baumeister, R. F. (1991). Identity crisis. In R. M. Lerner, A. C. Peterson, & J. Brooks-Gunn (Eds.), *Encyclopedia of adolescence* (Vol. 1). New York: Garland.

Becker, D. M., Yanek, L. R., Koffman, D. M., & Bronner, Y. C. (1999). Body image preferences among urban African Americans and whites from low income communities. *Ethnicity and Disease, 9*(3), 377–386.

Berghuis, J. P., Swift, W., Roffman, R. A., Stephens, R. S., & Copeland, J. (2006). The teen cannabis check-up: Exploring strategies for reaching young cannabis users. In R. A. Roffman & R. S. Stephens (Eds.), *Cannabis dependence: Its nature, consequences and treatment* (pp. 275–296). Cambridge, UK: Cambridge University Press.

Berg-Smith, S., Stevens, V., Brown, K., Van Horn, L., Gernhofer, N., Peters, E., et al. (1999). A brief motivational intervention to improve dietary adherence in adolescents. *Health Education Research, 14*(3), 399–410.

Birgden, A. (2004). Therapeutic jurisprudence and sex offenders: A psycho-legal approach to protection. *Sexual Abuse: A Journal of Research and Treatment, 16*, 351–364.

Blake, W., Turnbull, S., & Treasure, J. (1997). Stages and processes of change in eating disorders: Implications for therapy. *Clinical Psychology and Psychotherapy, 4*, 186–191.

Booth, K. M., Pinkston, M. M., & Poston, W. S. (2005). Obesity and the built environment. *Journal of the American Dietetic Association, 105*(5, Suppl. 1), S110–117.

Borsari, B., & Carey, K. (2001). Peer influences on college drinking: A review of the research. *Journal of Substance Abuse, 13*(4), 391–424.

Branstetter, S. A., Horn, K. A,. Dino, G., & Zhang, J. (2009). Beyond quitting: Predictors of teen smoking cessation reduction and acceleration following a school-based intervention. *Drug and Alcohol Dependence, 99*(1–3), 160–168.

Brehm, J. W. (1966). *A theory of psychological reactance.* New York: Academic Press.

Breslin, C., Li, S., Sdao-Jarvie, K., Tupker, E., & Ittig-Deland, V. (2002). Brief treatment for young substance abusers: A pilot study in an addiction treatment setting. *Psychology of Addictive Behaviors, 16,* 10–16.

Brown, R. A., Ramsey, S. E., Strong, D. R., Myers, M. G., Kahler, C. W., Lejuez, C. W., et al. (2003). Effects of motivational interviewing on smoking cessation in adolescents with psychiatric disorders. *Tobacco Control, 12.* (Suppl. 4), IV3–10.

Brug, J., Spikmans, F., Aartsen, C., Breedveld, B., Bes, R., & Ferieria, I. (2007). Training dieticians in basic motivational interviewing skills results in changes in their counseling style and lower saturated fat intake in their patients. *Journal of Nutrition Education and Behavior, 39,* 8–12.

Bryan, A., & Feldstein Ewing, S. W. (2008). *Alcohol use and sexual risk: An intervention* (1R01 AA013844). Rockville, MD: National Institute on Alcohol Abuse and Alcoholism.

Buckner, J. D., & Schmidt, N. B. (2008, November). *Motivational enhancement therapy increases CBT utilization among non-treatment seekers with social anxiety disorder.* Paper presented at the annual meeting of the Association for Behavioral and Cognitive Therapies, Orlando, FL.

Burke, B. L., Arkowitz, H., & Menchola, M. (2003). The efficacy of motivational interviewing: A meta-analysis of controlled clinical trials. *Journal of Consulting and Clinical Psychology, 71,* 843–861.

Carroll, K. M., Libby, B., Sheehan, J., & Hyland, N. (2001). Motivational interviewing to enhance treatment initiation in substance abusers: An effectiveness study. *American Journal on Addictions, 10,* 335–339.

Carroll, K. M., Sinha, R., & Easton, C. (2006). Engaging young probation-referred marijuana-abusing individuals in treatment. In R. A. Roffman & R. S. Stephens (Eds.), *Cannabis dependence. Its nature, consequences and treatment* (pp. 297–314). Cambridge, UK: Cambridge University Press.

Carroll, K. M., Easton, C. J., Nich, C., Hunkele, K. A., Neavins, T. M., Sinha, R., et al. (2006). The use of contigency management and motivational/skills building therapy to treat young adults with marijuana dependence. *Journal of Consulting and Clinical Psychology, 74,* 955–966.

Cassin, S. E., von Ranson, K. M., Heng, K. Y. W., Brar, J., & Wojtowicz, A. E. (2008). Adapted motivational interviewing for women with binge eating disorder: A randomized controlled trial. *Psychology of Addictive Behaviors, 22*(3), 417–425.

Centers for Disease Control and Prevention. (2007). *Sexually Transmitted Disease Surveillance.* Atlanta, GA: U.S. Department of Health and Human Services. Retrieved January 12, 2009, from *www.cdc.gov.std/stats 07/toc.htm.*

Centers for Disease Control and Prevention. (2006, June). Youth risk behavior surveillance survey. *MMWR, 55,* 69.

Centers for Disease Control and Prevention. (2008a). HIV/AIDS Fact Sheet: HIV/AIDS among Youth. Retrieved January 17, 2009, from *www.cdc.gov/hiv/resources/factsheets/PDF/youth.pdf.*

Centers for Disease Control and Prevention. (2008b). Youth Risk Behavior Surveillance Survey—United States, 2007. *MMWR, 57*(SS-4), 1–25.

Channon, S., Huws-Thomas, M. V., Gregory, J. W., & Rollnick, S. (2005). Motivational interviewing with teenagers with diabetes. *Clinical Child Psychology and Psychiatry, 10*, 43–51.

Channon, S., Huws-Thomas, M., Rollnick, S., Hood, K., Cannings-John, R., Rogers, C., et al. (2007). A multicenter randomized controlled trial of motivational interviewing in teenagers with diabetes. *Diabetes Care, 30*(6), 1390–1395.

Chapin, J. (2001). Self-protective pessimism: Optimistic bias in reverse. *North American Journal of Psychology, 3*, 253–262.

Chapin, J. R. (2000). Third-person perception and optimistic bias among urban minority at-risk youth. *Communication Research, 27*, 51–81.

Chen, K., Kandel, D. B., & Davies, M. (1997). Relationships between frequency and quantity of marijuana use and last year proxy dependence among adolescents and adults in the United States. *Drug and Alcohol Dependence, 46*(1–2), 53–67.

Chossis, I. C., Lance, C., Gache, P., Michaud, P. A., Pecoud, A., Rollnick, S., et al. (2007). Effect of training on primary care residents' performance in brief intervention: A randomized controlled trial. *Society of General Internal Medicine, 22*, 1144–1149.

Clark, H. W., Horton, A. M., Dennis, M., & Babor, T. F. (2002). Moving from research to practice just in time: The treatment of cannabis use disorders comes of age. *Addiction, 97*, 1–3.

Coffey, C., Carlin, J. B., Lynskey, M. T., Li, N., & Patton, G. C. (2003). Adolescent precursors of cannabis dependence: Findings from the Victorian Adolescent Health Cohort Study. *British Journal of Psychiatry, 182*(4), 330–336.

Colby, S. M., Monti, P. M., Barnett, N. P., Rohsenow, D. J., Weissman, K., Spirito, A., et al. (1998). Brief motivational interviewing in a hospital setting for adolescent smoking: A preliminary study. *Journal of Consulting and Clinical Psychology, 66*(3), 574–578.

Cole, D. A., Maxwell, S. E., Martin, J. M., Lachlin, G. P., Seroczynski, A. D., Tram, J. M., et al. (2001). The development of multiple domains of child and adolescent self-concept: A cohort sequential longitudinal design. *Child Development, 72*, 1723–1746.

Collins, W. A., & Laursen, B. (1992). Conflict and relationships during adolescence. In C. U. Shantz & W. W. Hartup (Eds.), *Conflict in child and adolescent development* (pp. 216–241). New York: Cambridge University Press.

Corrigan, P. (2004). How stigma interferes with mental health care. *American Psychologist, 59*, 614–625.

Crane, A. M., Roberts, M. E., & Treasure, J. (2007). Are obsessive-compulsive personality traits associated with a poor outcome in anorexia nervosa?: A systematic review of randomized controlled trials and naturalistic outcome studies. *International Journal of Eating Disorders, 40*(7), 581–588.

Currin, L., Schmidt, U., Treasure, J., & Jick, H. (2005). Time trends in eating disorder incidence. *British Journal of Psychiatry, 186*, 132–135.

Curry, S. J., Emery, S., Sporer, A. K., Mermelstein, R., Flay, B. R., Berbaum, M., et al. (2007). A national survey of tobacco cessation programs for youths. *American Journal of Public Health, 97*(1), 171–177.

Daly, M. (2006). *Engineering change: The impact of a collaborative training programme for graduate mentors to enhance motivation amongst vocational GCSE pupils.* Unpublished doctoral dissertation, University of Liverpool.

D'Amico, E. J., Osilla, K. C., & Hunter, S. B. (in press). Developing a group motivational interviewing intervention for adolescents at-risk for developing an alcohol or drug use disorder. *Alcoholism Treatment Quarterly.*

D'Amico, E. J. (2005). Factors that impact adolescents' intentions to utilize alcohol-related prevention services. *Journal of Behavioral Health Services and Research, 32,* 332–340.

D'Amico, E. J., Hunter, S., & Osilla, K. C. (2008). *Brief substance use intervention for youth in teen court* (R01DA019938). Rockville, MD: National Institute on Drug Abuse.

D'Amico, E. J., Miles, J. N. V., Stern, S. A., & Meredith, L. S. (2008). Brief motivational interviewing for teens at risk of substance use consequences: A randomized pilot study in a primary care clinic. *Journal of Substance Abuse Treatment, 35,* 53–61.

Davis, J. N., Kelly, L. A., Lane, C. J., Ventura, E. E., Byrd-Williams, C. E., Alexandar, K. A., et al. (2009). Randomized control trial to improve adiposity and insulin resistance in overweight Latino adolescents. *Obesity* (Silver Spring), 17(8), 1542–1548.

Davis, J. N., Tung, A., Chak, S. S., Ventura, E. E., Byrd-Williams, C. E., Alexander, K. E., et al. (2009). Aerobic and strength training reduces adiposity in overweight Latina adolescents. *Medicine and Science in Sports and Exercise, 41(7),* 1494–1503.

Davis, T. M., Baer, J. S., Saxon, A. J., & Kivlahan, D. R. (2003). Brief motivational feedback improves post-incarceration treatment contact among veterans with substance use disorders. *Drug and Alcohol Dependence, 69,* 197–203.

Dean, H., Touyz, S., Rieger, E., & Thornton, C. (2008). Group motivational enhancement therapy as an adjunct to inpatient treatment for eating disorders: A preliminary study. *European Eating Disorders Review, 16(4),* 256–267.

Deci, E. L., Koestner, R., & Ryan, R. M. (1999). A meta-analytical review of experiments examining the effects of extrinsic rewards on intrinsic motivation. *Psychological Bulletin, 125,* 627–668.

Deci, E. L., & Ryan, R. M. (1985). *Intrinsic motivation and self-determination in human behavior.* New York: Plenum Press.

Dennis, M. L., Dawud-Noursi, S., Muck, R., & McDermeit, M. (2003). The need for developing and evaluating adolescent treatment models. In S. J. Stevens & A. R. Morral (Eds.), *Adolescent substance abuse treatment in the United States: Exemplary models from a national evaluation study* (pp. 3–34). Binghamton, NY: Haworth Press.

Dennis, M., Godley, S. H., Diamond, G., Tims, F. M., Babor, T., Donaldson, J., et al. (2004). The cannabis youth treatment (CYT) study: Main findings from two randomized trials. *Journal of Substance Abuse Treatment, 27(3),* 197–213.

Diamond G., Leckrone J., Dennis M., & Godley, S. H. (2006). The cannabis youth treatment study: The treatment models and preliminary findings. In R. A. Roffman & R. S. Stephens (Eds.), *Cannabis dependence. Its nature, consequences and treatment* (pp. 247–274). Cambridge, UK: Cambridge University Press.

Dies, K. G. (2000). Adolescent development and a model of group psychotherapy: Effective leadership in the new millennium. *Journal of Child and Adolescent Group Therapy, 10*(2), 97–111.

Dishion, T. J., McCord, J., & Poulin, F. (1999). When interventions harm: Peer groups and problem behavior. *American Psychologist, 54*, 755–764.

Dishion, T. J., Shaw, D., Connell, A., Gardner, F., Weaver, C., & Wilson, M. (2008). The family check-up with high-risk indigent families: Preventing problem behavior by increasing parents' positive behavior support in early childhood. *Child Development, 79*, 1395–1414.

Dobbels, F., Vanhaecke, J., Desmyttere, A., Dupont, L., Nevens, F., & Geest, S. D. (2005). Prevalence and correlates of self-reported pretransplant nonadherence with medication in heart, liver, and lung transplant candidates. *Transplantation, 79*(11), 1588–1595.

Dodge, K. A., Dishion, T. J., & Lansford, J. E. (Eds.). (2006). *Deviant peer influences in programs for youth: Problems and Solutions.* New York: Guilford Press.

Drotar, D., & Ievers, C. (1994). Age difference in parent-child responsibilities for management of cystic fibrosis and insulin-dependent diabetes mellitus. *Developmental and Behavioral Pediatrics, 15*, 265–272.

Dubow, E. F., Lovko, K. R. J., & Kausch, D. F. (1990). Demographic differences in adolescents' health concerns and perceptions of helping agents. *Journal of Clinical Child Psychology, 19*, 44–54.

Dunn, E., Neighbors, C., & Larimer, M. (2006). Motivational enhancement therapy and self-help treatment for binge eaters. *Psychology of Addictive Behaviors, 20*(1), 44–52.

Eaton, D. K., Kann, L., Kinchen, S., Shanklin, S., Ross, J., Hawkins, J., et al. (2008). Youth risk behavior surveillance—United States, 2007. *MMWR Surveillance Summary, 57*(4), 1–131.

Ehrenreich, H., Rinn, T., Kunert, H. J., Moeller, M. R., Poser, W., Schilling, L., et al. (1999). Specific attentional dysfunction in adults following early start of cannabis use. *Psychopharmacology, 142*, 295–301.

Ellickson, P. L., & McGuigan, K. A. (2000). Early predictors of adolescent violence. *American Journal of Public Health, 90*, 566–572.

Emmons, K., & Rollnick, S. (2001). Motivational interviewing in health care settings: Opportunities and limitations. *American Journal of Preventive Medicine, 20*(1), 68–74.

Engle, B., Macgowan, M. J., Wagner, E. F., & Amrhein, P. (2010). Markers of marijuana use outcomes within adolescent substance abuse group treatment. *Research on Social Work Practice, 20*(3), 271–282.

Engle, D. E., & Arkowitz, H. (2006). *Ambivalence in psychotherapy: Facilitating readiness to change.* New York: Guilford Press.

Erickson, E. H. (1950). *Childhood and society.* New York: W. W. Norton.

Erickson, E. H. (1968). *Identity: Youth, and crisis.* New York: W. W. Norton.

Erickson, E. H. (1982). *The life cycle completed.* New York: W. W. Norton.

Erickson, S. J., Gerstle, M., & Feldstein, S. W. (2005). Brief interventions and motivational interviewing with children, adolescents, and their parents in pediatric health care settings: A review. *Archives of Pediatric Adolescent Medicine, 159*, 1173–1180.

Feld, R., Woodside, D. B., Kaplan, A. S., Olmsted, M. P., & Carter, J. C. (2001). Pretreatment motivational enhancement therapy for eating disorders: A pilot study. *International Journal of Eating Disorders, 29*(4), 393–400.

Feldstein Ewing, S. W., Hendrickson, S., & Payne, N. (2008). The validity of the desired effects of drinking scale with a late adolescent sample. *Motivational Interviewing in Groups, 22*(4), 587–591.

Feldstein Ewing, S. W., Walters, S., & Baer, J. S. (in press). Approaching group MI with adolescents and young adults: Strengthening the developmental fit. In C. C. I. Wagner & K. S. Ingersoll (Eds.), *Motivational interviewing in groups.* New York: Guilford Press.

Feldstein, S. W., & Ginsburg, J. I. D. (2006). Motivational interviewing with dually diagnosed adolescents in juvenile justice settings. *Brief Treatment and Crisis Intervention, 6,* 218–233.

Feldstein, S. W., & Ginsburg, J. I. D. (2007). Sex, drugs, and rock 'n' rolling with resistance: Motivational interviewing in juvenile justice settings. In A. R. Roberts & D. W. Springer (Eds.), *Handbook of forensic mental health with victims and offenders: Assessment, treatment, and research* (pp. 247–271). New York: Charles C. Thomas.

Fergusson, D. M., Horwood, L. J., & Swain-Campbell, N. (2002). Cannabis use and psychosocial adjustment in adolescence and young adulthood. *Addiction, 97*(9), 1123–1135.

Fisher, W. A, Fisher, J. D. & Harman, J. J. (2003). The information–motivation–behavioral skills model: A general social psychological approach to understanding and promoting health behavior. In J. Suls & K. Wallston (Eds.), *Social psychological foundations of health* (pp. 82–106). London: Blackwell.

Flores, P. J., & Mahon, L. (1993). The treatment of addiction in group psychotherapy. *International Journal of Group Psychotherapy, 43*(2), 143–156.

Foltz, C., Overton, W. F., & Ricco, R. B. (1995). Proof construction: Adolescent development from inductive to deductive problem-solving strategies. *Journal of Experimental Child Psychology, 59,* 179–195.

Ford, J. A. (2005). Substance use, the social bond, and delinquency. *Sociological Inquiry, 75,* 109–128.

Freeman, A., & McCloskey, R. D. (2003). Impediments to effective psychotherapy. In R. L. Leahy (Ed.), *Roadblocks in cognitive-behavioral therapy: Transforming challenges into opportunities for change* (pp. 24–48). New York: Guilford Press.

Gance-Cleveland, B. (2005). Motivational interviewing as a strategy to increase families' adherence to treatment regimens. *Journal of Special Pediatric Nursing, 10,* 151–155.

Ginsburg, J. I. D. (2000). *Using motivational interviewing to enhance treatment readiness in offenders with symptoms of alcohol dependence.* Unpublished doctoral dissertation, Carleton University, Ottawa, Ontario, Canada.

Ginsburg, J. I. D., Mann, R. E., Rotgers, F., & Weekes, J. R. (2002). Motivational interviewing with criminal justice populations. In W. R. Miller & S. Rollnick (Eds.), *Motivational interviewing: Preparing people for change* (2nd ed., 333–346). New York: Guilford Press.

Glasgow, R. E., Goldstein, M. G., Ockene, J. K., & Pronk, N. P. (2004). Translating what we have learned into practice: Principles and hypotheses for interventions addressing multiple behaviors in primary care. *American Journal of Preventive Medicine, 27*(2, Suppl. 1), 88–101.

Glasgow, R. E., Vogt, T. M., & Boles, S. M. (1999). Evaluating the public health impact of health promotion interventions: The re-aim framework. *American Journal of Public Health, 89*(9), 1322–1327.

Goldberg, D., Hoffman, A., Farinha, M., Marder, D. C., Tinson Mitchem, L., Burton, D., et al. (1994). Physician delivery of smoking-cessation advice based on the stages-of-change model. *American Journal of Preventive Medicine, 10*, 267–274.

Gollwitzer, P. M. (1999). Implementation Intentions: Strong effects of simple plans. *American Psychologist, 54*, 493–503.

Goran, M. I. (2001). Metabolic precursors and effects of obesity in children: A decade of progress, 1990–1999. *American Journal of Clinical Nutrition, 73*(2), 158–171.

Goran, M. I., Reynolds, K. D., & Lindquist, C. H. (1999). Role of physical activity in the prevention of obesity in children. *International Journal of Obesity and Related Metabolic Disorders: Journal of the International Association for the Study of Obesity, 23*(Suppl. 3), S18–33.

Gordon-Larsen, P., Adair, L. S., & Popkin, B. M. (2002). Ethnic differences in physical activity and inactivity patterns and overweight status. *Obesity Research, 10*(3), 141–149.

Gortmaker, S. L., Must, A., Perrin, J. M., Sobol, A. M., & Dietz, W. H. (1993). Social and economic consequences of overweight in adolescence and young adulthood. *New England Journal of Medicine, 329*(14), 1008–1012.

Gowers, S., Clark, A., Roberts, C., Griffiths, A., Edwards, V., Bryan, C., et al. (2007). Clinical effectiveness of treatments for anorexia nervosa in adolescents: randomised controlled trial. *British Journal of Psychiatry, 191*, 427–435.

Gowers, S. G., Smyth, B., & Shore, A. (2004). The impact of a motivational assessment interview on initial response to treatment in adolescent anorexia nervosa. *European Eating Disorder Review, 12*, 87–93.

Graham, A. W., & Fleming, M. S. (1998). *Brief interventions* (2nd ed.). Chevy Chase, MD: American Society of Addictive Medicine.

Gray, E., McCambridge, J., & Strang, J. (2005). The effectiveness of motivational interviewing delivered by youth workers in reducing drinking, cigarette and cannabis smoking among young people: Quasi-experimental pilot study. *Alcohol and Alcoholism, 40*, 535–539.

Greene, K., Krcmar, M., Walters, L. H., Rubin, D. L., & Hale, J. L. (2000). Targeting adolescent risk-taking behaviors: The contributions of egocentrism and sensation-seeking. *Journal of Adolescence, 23*(4), 439–461.

Greenwald, R. (2002). Motivation-Adaptive Skills-Trauma Resolution (MASTR) therapy for adolescents with conduct problems: An open trial. *Journal of Aggression, Maltreatment and Trauma, 6*, 237–261.

Grimshaw, G. M., & Stanton, A. (2006). Tobacco cessation interventions for young people. *Cochrane Database of Systematic Reviews*, Issue 4 (Article no. CD003289), DOI: 10.1002/14651858.CD003289.pub4.

Haigh, R., & Treasure, J. (2003). Investigating the needs of carers in the area of eating disorders: development of the Carers' Needs Assessment Measure (CaNAM). *European Eating Disorders Review, 11*, 125–141.

Hall, J. A., Smith, D. C., & Williams, J. K. (2008). Strengths Oriented Family Therapy (SOFT): A manual-guided treatment for substance-involved teens and their families. In C. W. LeCroy (Ed.), *Handbook of evidence-based treatment manuals for children and adolescents* (2nd ed.) New York: Oxford University Press.

Harper, R., & Hardy, S. (2000). An evaluation of motivational interviewing as a method of intervention with clients in a probation setting. *British Journal of Social Work, 30*, 393–400.

Harris, E. C., & Barraclough, B. (1998). Excess mortality of mental disorder. *British Journal of Psychiatry, 173*, 11–53.

Hawkins, J., Graham, J., Maquin, E., Abbott, R., Hill, R., & Catalano, R. (1997). Exploring the effects of age and alcohol use initiation and psychosocial risk factors on subsequent alcohol misuse. *Journal of Studies on Alcohol, 58*, 280–290.

Hayatbakhsh, M. R., Najman, J. M., Jamrozik, K., Mamun, A. A., Alati, R., & Bor, W. (2007). Cannabis and anxiety and depression in young adults: A large prospective study. *Journal of the American Academy of Child and Adolescent Psychiatry, 46*(3), 408–417.

Hettema, J., Steele, J., & Miller, W. R. (2005). Motivational interviewing. *Annual Review of Clinical Psychology, 1*(1), 91–111.

Hickman, G. P., Bartholomew, M., & Mathwig, J. (2008). Differential developmental pathways of high school dropouts and graduates. *Journal of Educational Research, 102*, 3–14.

Holmbeck, G. N. (1996). A model of family relational transformations during the transition to adolescence: Parent-adolescent conflict and adaptation. In J. A. Graber, J. Brooks-Gunn, & A. C. Petersen (Eds.), *Transitions through adolescence: Interpersonal domains and context* (pp. 167–199). Mahwah, NJ: Erlbaum.

Holmbeck, G. N., O'Mahar, K. O., Abad, M., Colder, C., & Updegrove, A. (2006). Cognitive-behavioral therapy with adolescents: Guides from developmental psychology. In P. C. Kendall (Ed.), *Child and adolescent therapy: Cognitive-behavioral procedures (3rd ed.)*, (pp. 419–464). New York: Guilford Press.

Hong, S.-M., Giannakopoulos, E., Laing, D., & Williams, N. A. (1994). Psychological reactance: Effects of age and gender, *Journal of Social Psychology, 134*(2), 223–228.

Horn, K., Dino, G., Goldcamp, J., Kalsekar, I., & Mody, R. (2005). The impact of not on tobacco on teen smoking cessation: End-of-program evaluation results, 1998 to 2003. *Journal of Adolescent Research, 20*(6), 640–661.

Horn, K., Dino, G., Hamilton, C., & Noerachmanto, N. (2007). Efficacy of an emergency department-based motivational teenage smoking intervention. *Preventing Chronic Disease, 4*(1), A08.

Horn, K., Dino, G., Hamilton, C., Noerachmanto, N., & Zhang, J. (2008). Feasibility of a smoking cessation intervention for teens in the emergency department: Reach, implementation fidelity, and acceptability. *American Journal of Critical Care, 17*(3), 205–216.

Horn, K., Fernandes, A., Dino, G., Massey, C., & Kalsekar, I. (2003). Adolescent nicotine dependence and smoking cessation outcomes. *Addictive Behaviors, 28*, 769–776.

Ingersoll, K. S., Ceperich, S. D., Nettleman, M. D., Karanda, K., Brocksen, S., & Johnson, B. A. (2005). Reducing alcohol-exposed pregnancy risk in college women: Initial outcomes of a clinical trial of a motivational intervention. *Journal of Substance Abuse Treatment, 29*(3), 173–180.

Ingersoll, K. S., Wagner, C. C., & Gharib, S. (2006). *Motivational groups for community substance abuse programs* (3rd ed.). Rockville, MD: Substance Abuse Mental Health Services Administration.

Jelalian, E., Boergers, J., Alday, C. S., & Frank, R. (2003). Survey of physician attitudes and practices related to pediatric obesity. *Clinical Pediatrics, 42*(3), 235–245.

Jemal, A., Chu, K. C., & Tarone, R. E. (2001). Recent trends in lung cancer mortality in the United States. *Journal of the National Cancer Institute, 93*(4), 277–283.

Jessor, R. (1992). Risk behavior in adolescence: A psychosocial framework for understanding and action. *Developmental Review, 12*(4), 374–390.

Johnson, S. D., Stiffman, A., Hadley-Ives, E., & Elze, D. (2001). An analysis of stressors and co-morbid mental health problems that contribute to youths' paths to substance-specific services. *Journal of Behavioral Health Services and Research, 4*, 412–426.

Johnston, L. D., O'Malley, P. M., Bachman, J. G., & Schulenberg, J. E. (2008). *Monitoring the Future national survey results on drug use, 1975–2007: Volume 1, Secondary school students* (NIH Publication No. 08-6418A). Bethesda, MD: National Institute on Drug Abuse.

Juszczak, L., Melinkovich, P., & Kaplan, D. (2003). Use of health and mental health services by adolescents across multiple delivery sites. *Journal of Adolescent Health, 32*, 108–118.

Kaminer, Y. (2005). Challenges and opportunities of group therapy for adolescent substance abuse: A critical review. *Addictive Behaviors, 30*(9), 1765–1774.

Kaminer, Y., Burleson, J. A., & Goldberger, R. (2002). Cognitive-behavioral coping skills and psychoeducation therapies for adolescent substance abuse. *Journal of Nervous and Mental Disease, 190*, 737–745.

Karno, M. P., & Longabaugh, R. (2004). What do we know?: Process analysis and the search for a better understanding of Project MATCH's anger-by-treatment matching effect. *Journal of Studies on Alcohol, 65*, 501–512.

Kavanagh, D. J., Young, R., White, A., Saunders, J. B., Wallis, J., Shockley, N., et al. (2004). A brief motivational intervention for substance misuse in recent-onset psychosis. *Drug and Alcohol Review, 23*(2), 151–155.

Kelly, A. B., & Lapworth, K. (2006). The HYP program—Targeted motivational interviewing for adolescent violations of school tobacco policy. *Preventive Medicine, 43*, 466–471.

Kilmer, J. R., Walker, D. D., Lee, C. M., Palmer, R. S., Mallett, K. A., Fabiano, P., et al. (2006). Misperceptions of college student marijuana use: Implications for prevention. *Journal of Studies on Alcohol, 67*(2), 277–281.

Kimm, S. Y., Barton, B. A., Berhane, K., Ross, J. W., Payne, G. H., & Schreiber,

G. B. (1997). Self-esteem and adiposity in black and white girls: the NHLBI Growth and Health Study. *Annals of Epidemiology, 7*(8), 550–560.

Kipke, M. D., Iverson, E., Moore, D., Booker, C., Ruelas, V., Peters, A. L., et al. (2007). Food and park environments: Neighborhood-level risks for childhood obesity in East Los Angeles. *Journal of Adolescent Health, 40*(4), 325–333.

Kokkevi, A., Nic Gabhainn, S., & Spyropoulou, M. (2006). Early initiation of *cannabis* use: A cross-national European perspective. *Journal of Adolescent Health, 39*, 712–719.

Kolagotla, L., & Adams, W. (2004). Ambulatory management of childhood obesity. *Obesity Research, 12*(2), 275–283.

Kuczmarski, R. J., Ogden, C. L., Guo, S. S., et al. (2002). 2000 CDC growth charts for the United States: Methods and development. *Vital Health Statistics, 11*(246).

LaBrie, J. W., Pedersen, E. R., Thompson, A. D., & Earleywine, M. (2008). A brief decisional balance intervention increases motivation and behavior regarding condom use in high-risk heterosexual college men. *Archives of Sexual Behavior, 37*(2), 330–339.

La Greca, A. M., & Shulman, W. B. (1995). Adherence to prescribed medical regimens. In M. C. Roberts (Ed.), *Handbook of pediatric psychology* (2nd ed., pp. 119–140). New York: Guilford Press.

Laird, R. D., Pettit, G. S., Bates, J. E., & Dodge, K. A. (2003). Parents' monitoring-relevant knowledge and adolescents' delinquent behavior: Evidence of correlated developmental changes and reciprocal influences *Child Development, 74*(3), 752–768.

Lambert, M. J., & Barley, D. E. (2001). Research summary on the therapeutic relationship and psychotherapy outcome. *Psychotherapy: Theory, Research, Practice, Training, 38*,357–361.

Landowski, L. A. (1998). A motivational intervention for adolescent smokers. *Preventive Medicine, 27*, A39–A46.

Lane, C., Johnson, S., Rollnick, S., Edwards, K., & Lyons, M. (2003). Consulting about lifestyle change: Evaluation of a training course for diabetes nurses. *Practicing Diabetes International, 20*, 204–208.

Lepper, M. R., Corpus, J. H., & Iyengar, S. S. (2005). Intrinsic and extrinsic motivational orientations in the classroom. *Journal of Educational Psychology, 97*, 184–196.

Lewis, L. B., Sloane, D. C., Nascimento, L. M., Diamant, A. L., Guinyard, J. J., Yancey, A. K., et al. (2005). African Americans' access to healthy food options in South Los Angeles restaurants. *American Journal of Public Health, 95*(4), 668–673.

Lewis, M. A., & Neighbors, C. (2006). Social norms approaches using descriptive drinking norms education: A review of the research. *Journal of American College Health, 54*, 213–218.

Lobstein, T., Baur, L., & Uauy, R. (2004). *Obesity in children and young people: A crisis in public health.* London: IASO International Obesity Task Force.

Loeber, R., & Farrington, D. P. (2000). Young children who commit crime: Epidemiology, developmental origins, risk factors, early interventions, and policy implications. *Development and Psychopathology, 12*, 737–762.

López, C. (2008). *An examination of central coherence in eating disorders and its clinical implications.* Unpublished manuscript, Kings College London.

López, C., Roberts, M. E., Tchanturia, K., & Treasure, J. (2008). Using neuropsychological feedback therapeutically in treatment for anorexia nervosa: Two illustrative case reports. *European Eating Disorders Review, 16*(6), 411–420.

López, C., Tchanturia, K., Stahl, D., & Treasure, J. (2008). Central coherence in eating disorders: A systematic review. *Psychological Medicine, 38*(10), 1393–1404.

Lowe, S., Zipfel, S., Buchholz, C., Dupont, Y., Reas, D., & Herzog, W. (2001). Long-term outcome of anorexia in a prospective 21-year follow-up study. *Psychological Medicine, 31*, 881–890.

Lunkenheimer, E. S., Dishion, T. J., Shaw, D. S., Connell, A. M., Gardner, F., Wilson, M. N., et al. (2008). Collateral benefits of the Family Check-Up on early childhood school readiness: Indirect effects of parents' positive behavior support. *Developmental Psychology, 44*, 1737–1752.

MacDonell, K., Naar-King, S., Murphy, D. A., Parsons, J., & Harper, G. (2010). Predictors of medication adherence in high risk youth living with HIV. *Journal of Pediatric Psychology, 35*, 593–601.

MacLennan, B. W., & Dies, K. R. (1992). *Group counseling and psychotherapy with adolescents* (2nd ed.). New York: Columbia University Press.

Malekoff, A. (2004). *Group work with adolescents: Principles and practice* (2nd ed.). New York: Guilford Press.

Maltby, N., & Tolin, D. F. (2005). A brief motivational intervention for treatment-refusing OCD patients. *Cognitive Behavior Therapy, 34*, 176–184.

Mann, R. E., Ginsberg, J. I. D., & Weeks, J. R. (2002). Motivational interviewing with offenders. In M. McMurran (Ed.), *Motivating offenders to change: A guide to enhancing engagement in therapy.* Hove, West Sussex, UK: Wiley.

March, J. S., Franklin, M., Nelson, A., & Foa, E. (2001). Cognitive-behavioral therapy for pediatric obsessive-compulsive disorder. *Journal of Clinical Child Psychology, 30*, 8–18.

Marlatt, G. A., Larimer, M. E., Baer, J. S., & Quigley, L. A. (1993). Harm reduction for alcohol problems: Moving beyond the controlled drinking controversy. *Behavior Therapy, 24*, 461–504.

Martin, G. & Copeland, J. (2008). The adolescent cannabis check-up: Randomized trial of a brief intervention for young *cannabis* users. *Journal of Substance Abuse Treatment, 34*, 407–414.

Martino, S., Ball, S. A., Gallon, S. L., Hall, D., Garcia, M., Ceperich, S., et al. (2006). *Motivational interviewing assessment: supervisory tools for enhancing proficiency.* Salem: Northwest Frontier Addiction Technology Transfer Center, Oregon Health and Science University.

Martino, S., Carroll, K., Kostas, D., Perkins, J., & Rounsaville, B.(2002). Dual diagnosis motivational interviewing: A modification of motivational interviewing for substance-abusing patients with psychotic disorders. *Journal of Substance Abuse Treatment, 23*, 297–308.

Martino, S., Carroll, K. M., O'Malley, S. S., & Rounsaville, B. J. (2000). Motivational interviewing with psychiatrically ill substance abusing patients. *American Journal on Addictions, 9*, 88–91.

Martino, S., Haesler, F., Belitsky, R., Pantalon, M., & Fortin, A. H. (2007). Teaching brief motivational interviewing to year three medical students. *Medical Education, 41*, 16–167.

McCambridge, J., Slym, R. L., & Strang J. (2008). RCT of motivational interviewing compared with drug information and advice for early intervention among young cannabis users. *Addiction, 103*, 1809–1818.

McCambridge, J., & Strang, J. (2004). The efficacy of single-session motivational interviewing in reducing drug consumption and perceptions of drug-related risks and harm among young people: Results from a multi-site cluster randomized trial. *Addiction, 99*, 39–52.

McCambridge, J., & Strang, J. (2005). Deterioration over time in effect of motivational interviewing in reducing drug consumption and related risk among young people. *Addiction, 100*, 470–478.

McClelland G. M., Elkington, K. S., Teplin, L. A., & Abram, K. M. (2004). Multiple substance use disorders in juvenile detainees. *Journal of the American Academy of Child and Adolescent Psychiatry, 43*, 1215–1224.

McDonald, P., Colwell, B., Backinger, C., Husten, C., & Maule, C. (2003). Better practices for youth tobacco cessation: Evidence of review panel. *American Journal of Health Behavior, 27*(Suppl. 2), S144–S158.

Melnick, G., De Leon, G., Hawke, J., Jainchill, N. & Kressel, D. (1997). Motivational and readiness for therapeutic community treatment among adolescents and adult substance abusers. *American Journal of Drug and Alcohol Abuse, 23*, 485–506.

Merlo, L. J., Storch, E. A., Lehmkuhl, H. D., Jacob, M. L., Murphy, T. K., Goodman, W. K., et al. (2010). Cognitive-behavioral therapy plus motivational interviewing improves outcome for pediatric obsessive–compulsive disorder: A preliminary study. *Cognitive Behaviour Therapy, 39*, 24–27.

Mermelstein, R. (2003). Teen smoking cessation. *Tobacco Control, 12*(Suppl. 1), i25–i34.

Mermelstein, R., & Turner, L. (2006). Web-based support as an adjunct to group-based smoking cessation for adolescents. *Nicotine and Tobacco Research, 8*(Suppl. 1), S69–76.

Merriam-Webster Online Dictionary. Retrieved September 1, 2009, from *www.merriam-webster.com/dictionary/empathy*

Merten, D. E. (1996). Visibility and vulnerability: Responses to rejection by nonaggressive junior high school boys. *Journal of Early Adolescence, 16*, 5–26.

Meynard, A. (2008). *Health Behavior changes with adolescents and young people in various settings.* Paper presented at the International Conference on Motivational Interviewing.

Milgrom, H., Bender, B., Ackerson, L., Bowry, P., Smith, B., & Rand, C. (1996). Noncompliance and treatment failure in Children with asthma. *Journal of Allergy and Clinical Immunology, 98*, 1051–1057.

Miller, W. R. (1983). Motivational interviewing with problem drinkers. *Behavioural Psychotherapy, 11*, 147–172.

Miller, W. R. (2008). It all depends. *Addiction, 11*, 1819–1820.

Miller, W. R., Hendrickson, S. M. L., Venner, K., Bisono, M. S., Daughtery, M., & Yahne, C. E. (2008). Cross-cultural training in motivational interviewing. *Journal of Teaching the Addictions, 7*(1), 4–15.

Miller, W. R., & Mount, K. (2001). A small study of training in motivational interviewing: Does one workshop change clinician and client behavior? *Behavioural and Cognitive Psychotherapy, 29*, 457–471.

Miller, W. R., & Mount, K. A. (2005). A small study of training in motivational interviewing: Does one workshop change clinician and client behavior? *Behavioural and Cognitive Psychotherapy, 29*, 457–471.

Miller, W. R., Moyers, T. B. Ernst, D., & Amrhein, P. (2003, November.). *Manual for the Motivational Interviewing Skill Code (MISC) V. 2.0.* Retrieved June 2010 from *www.motivationalinterviewing.org/training/misc2.pdf.*

Miller, W. R., & Rollnick, S. (2002). *Motivational interviewing: Preparing people for change* (2nd ed.). New York: Guilford Press.

Miller, W. R., & Rollnick, S. (2009). Ten things that motivational interviewing is not. *Behavioural and Cognitive Psychotherapy, 37*, 129–140.

Miller, W. R., & Rose, G. S. (2009). Toward a theory of motivational interviewing. *American Psychologist, 64*, 527–537.

Miller, W. R., & Sanchez, V. C. (1994). Motivating young adults for treatment and lifestyle change. In G. Howard (Ed.), *Issues in alcohol use and misuse by young adults* (pp. 55–82). Notre Dame, IN: University of Notre Dame Press.

Miller, W. R., Sorensen, J. L., Selzer, J. A., & Brigham, G. S. (2006). Disseminating evidence-based practices in substance abuse treatment: A review with suggestions. *Journal of Substance Abuse Treatment, 31*, 25–39.

Miller, W. R., Villanueva, M., Tonigan, J. S., & Cuzmar, I. (2007). Are special treatments needed for special populations? *Alcoholism Treatment Quarterly, 25*(4), 63–78.

Miller, W. R., Yahne, C. E., Moyers, T. B., Martinez, J., & Pirritano, M. (2004). A randomized trial of methods to help clinicians learn motivational interviewing. *Journal of Consulting and Clinical Psychology, 72*, 1050–1062.

Milton, M. H., Maule, C. O., Backinger, C. L., & Gregory, D. M.(2003). Recommendations and guidance for practice in youth tobacco cessation. *American Journal of Health Behavior, 27*(Suppl. 2), S159–169.

Monti, P. M., Colby, S. M., Barnett, N. P., Spirito, A., Rohsenow, D. J., Myers, M., et al. (1999). Brief intervention for harm reduction with alcohol-positive older adolescents in a hospital emergency department. *Journal of Consulting and Clinical Psychology, 67*, 989–994.

Moore, S., & Parsons, J. A. (2000). A research agenda for adolescent risk-taking: Where do we go from here? *Journal of Adolescence, 23*, 371–376.

Moos, R. H. (2007). Theory-based active ingredients of effective treatments for substance use disorders. *Drug and Alcohol Dependence, 88*, 109–121.

Morris, A. D., Boyle, D. I., McMahon, A. D., Greene, S. A., MacDonald, T. M., & Newton, R. W. (1997). Adherence to insulin treatment, glycemic control, and ketoacidosis in insulin-dependent diabetes mellitus. *Lancet, 350*(9090), 1505–1510.

Moyers, T. B., Manuel, J. K., Wilson, P. G., Hendrickson, S. M. L., Talcot, W., & Durand, P. (2008). A randomized trial investigating training in motivational interviewing for behavioral health providers. *Behavioural and Cognitive Psychotherapy, 36*, 149–162.

Moyers, T., Martin, M., Catley, D., Harris, K. J., & Ahluwalia, J. S. (2003). Assessing the integrity of motivational interviewing interventions. *Behavioural and Cognitive Psychotherapy, 31*, 177–184.

Moyers, T. B., Martin, T., Manuel, J. K., Hendrickson, S. M., & Miller, W. R. (2005). Assessing competence in the use of motivational interviewing. *Journal of Substance Abuse Treatment, 28*(19–26).

Mueller, U., Sokol, B., & Overton, W. F. (1999). Developmental sequences in class reasoning and propositional reasoning. *Journal of Experimental Child Psychology, 74*, 69–106.

Naar-King, S., Arfken, C., Frey, M., Harris, M., Secord, E., & Ellis, D. (2006). Psychosocial factors and treatment adherence in pediatric HIV/AIDS. *AIDS Care, 18*, 621–628.

Naar-King, S., Lam, P., Wang, B., Wright, K., Parsons, J. T., & Frey, M. A. (2008). Brief report: Maintenance of effects of motivational enhancement therapy to improve risk behaviors and HIV-related health in a randomized controlled trial of youth living with HIV. *Journal of Pediatric Psychology, 33*(4), 441–445.

Naar-King, S., Outlaw, A., Green-Jones, M., & Wright, K. (2009). Motivational interviewing by peer outreach workers: A pilot randomized clinical trial to retain adolescents and young adults in HIV care. *AIDS Care, 21*, 866–873.

Naar-King, S., Parsons, J. T., Murphy, D. A., Chen, X., Harris, R., Belzer, M. et al. (2009). Improving health outcomes for youth living with HIV. A multisite randomized trial of a motivational intervention targeting multiple risk behaviors. *Archives of Pediatrics and Adolescent Medicine, 163*(12), 1092–1098.

Naar-King, S., Templin, T., Wright, K., Frey, M., Parsons, J. T., & Lam, P. (2006). Psychosocial factors and medication adherence in HIV positive youth. *AIDS Patient Care and STDs, 20*, 44–47.

Nagamune, N., & Bellis, J. M. (2002). Decisional balance of condom use and depressed mood among incarcerated male adolescents. *Acta Medica Okayama, 56*(6), 287–294.

Narayan, K. M., Boyle, J. P., Thompson, T. J., Sorensen, S. W., & Williamson, D. F. (2003). Lifetime risk for diabetes mellitus in the United States. *Journal of the American Medical Association, 290*(14), 1884–1890.

Nation, M., Crusto, C., Wandersman, A., Kumpfer, K. L., Seybolt, D., Morrissey-Kane, E., et al. (2003). What works in prevention: Principles of effective prevention programs. *American Psychologist, 58*, 449–456.

National Institute for Clinical Excellence. (2004). *National Clinical Practice Guideline: Eating Disorders: Core interventions in the treatment and management of anorexia nervosa, bulimia nervosa, and related eating disorders.* London: Author.

Nickoletti, P., & Taussig, H. N. (2006). Outcome expectancies and risk behaviors in maltreated adolescents. *Journal of Research on Adolescence, 16*, 217–228.

Nissen, K. B. (2006). Effective adolescent substance abuse treatment in juvenile justice settings: practice and policy recommendations. *Child and Adolescent Social Work Journal, 23*(3), 298–315.

Nock, M. K. & Ferriter, C. (2005). Parent management of attendance and adherence in child and adolescent therapy: A conceptual and empirical review. *Clinical Child and Family Psychology Review, 8*, 149–166.

Nock, M. K. & Kazdin, A. E. (2005). Randomized controlled trial of a brief intervention for increasing participation in parent management training. *Journal Consulting Clinical Psychology, 73*, 872–879.

Northen, H., & Kurland, R. (2001). Social work with groups (3rd ed.) [Book review]. *Social Work with Groups, 24*(3–4), 173–175.

Office of Health Economics. (1994). *Eating disorders.* London: Author.

Ogden, C. L., Carroll, M. D., & Flegal, K. M. (2008). High body mass index for age among US children and adolescents, 2003–2006. *Journal of the American Medical Association, 299*(20), 2401–2405.

Ogden, C., Yanovski, S., Carroll, M., & Flegal, K. (2007). The epidemiology of obesity. *Gastroenterology, 132*(6), 2087–2102.

Osborn, C. J. (2004). Seven salutary suggestions for counselor stamina. *Journal of Counseling and Development, 82*, 319–328.

Otto-Salaj, L. L., Gore-Felton, C., McGarvey, E., & Canterbury II, R. J. (2002). Psychiatric functioning and substance use: Factors associated with HIV risk among incarcerated adolescents. *Child Psychiatry and Human Development, 33*(2), 91–106.

Outlaw, A., Naar-King, S., Green-Jones, M., Wright, K., Condon, K., & Sherry, L. (in press). Predictors of retention in HIV care youth living with HIV: A prospective study. *Journal of Pediatric Psychology.*

Outlaw, A., Naar-King, S., Parsons, J. T., Green-Jones, M. & Secord, E. (2010). Using motivational interviewing in HIV field outreach with young African American men who have sex with men: A randomized clinical trial. *American Journal of Public Health, 100*(Supp. 1), S146–151.

Park, M. J., Mulye, T. P., Adams, S., Brindis, C., & Irwin, C. (2006). The health status of young adults in the United States. *Journal of Adolescent Health, 39*, 305–317.

Parker, J. G., & Asher, S. R. (1987). Peer relations and later personal adjustment: Are low-accepted children at risk? *Psychological Bulletin, 102*, 357–389.

Parsons, J. T., Rosof, E., Punzalan, J. C., & Di Maria, L. (2005). Integration of motivational interviewing and cognitive behavioral therapy to improve HIV medication adherence and reduce substance use among HIV-positive men and women: Results of a pilot project. *AIDS Patient Care and STDs, 19*, 31–39.

Parsons, J. T., Siegel, A. W., & Cousins, J. H. (1997). Late adolescent risk-taking: Effects of perceived benefits and perceived risks on behavioral intentions and behavioral change. *Journal of Adolescence, 20*, 381–392.

Perdue, T., Hagan, H., Thiede, H., & Valleroy, L. (2003). Depression and HIV risk behavior among Seattle-area injection drug users and young men who have sex with men. *AIDS Education and Prevention, 15*, 81–92.

Perkins-Dock, R. E. (2001). Family interventions with incarcerated youth: A review of the literature. *International Journal of Offender Therapy and Comparative Criminology, 45*, 606–625.

Perrin, E. M., Finkle, J. P., & Benjamin, J. T. (2007). Obesity prevention and the primary care pediatrician's office. *Current Opinion Pediatrics, 19*, 354–361.

Perrin, E. M., Flower, K. B., Garrett, J., & Ammerman, A. S. (2005). Preventing and treating obesity: pediatricians' self-efficacy, barriers, resources, and advocacy. *Ambulatory Pediatrics, 5*(3), 150–156.

Peterson, A. V., Kealey, K. A., Mann, S. L., Marek, P. M., Ludman, E. J., Liu,

J., et al. (2009). Group-randomized trial of a proactive, personalized telephone counseling intervention for adolescent smoking cessation. *Journal of the National Cancer Institute, 101*, 1378–1392.

Piaget, J. (1967). *Six psychological studies* (A. Tenzer & D. Elkind, Trans.). New York: Random House.

Piaget, J. (1971). The theory of stages in cognitive development. In Dr. R. Green (Ed.), *Measurement and Piaget*. New York: McGraw-Hill.

Piaget, J. (1972). Intellectual evolution from adolescence to adulthood. *Human Development, 15*, 1012.

Picciano, J. F., Roffman, R. A., Kalichman, S. C., Rutledge, S. E., & Berghuis, J. P. (2001). A telephone based brief intervention using motivational enhancement to facilitate HIV risk reduction among MSM: A pilot study. *AIDS and Behavior, 5*, 251–262.

Piper, W. E., & McCallum, M. (1994). Selection of patients for group interventions. In H. S. Bernard & K. R. MacKenzie (Eds.), *Basics of group psychotherapy*. New York: Guilford Press.

Pope, H., Gruber, A., Hudson, J., Cohane, G., Huestis, M., & Yurgelun-Todd, D. (2003). Early-onset cannabis use and cognitive deficits: what is the nature of the association? *Drug and Alcohol Dependence, 69*(3), 303–310.

Prochaska, J. O., & DiClemente, C. C. (1984). *The transtheoretical approach: crossing traditional boundaries of therapy*. Homewood, IL: Dow/Jones Irwin.

Prochaska, J. O., DiClemente, C. C., & Norcross, J. C. (1992). In search of how people change. *American Psychologist, 47*(9), 1102–1114.

Prochaska J. O., Velicer, W. F., Rossi, J. S., Goldstein, M. G., Marcus, B. H., Rakowski, W., et al. (1994). Stages of change and decisional balance for 12 problem behaviors. *Health Psychology, 19*, 39–46.

Prokhorov, A. V., Winickoff, J. P., Ahluwalia, J. S., Ossip-Klein, D., Tanski, S., Lando, H. A., et al. (2006). Youth tobacco use: A global perspective for child health care clinicians. *Pediatrics, 118*(3), e890–903.

Public Agenda. (1999). *Kids these days '99: What Americans really think about the next generation*. New York: Author.

Purdon, C., Rowa, K., & Antony, M. M. (2004). Treatment fears in individuals awaiting treatment of OCD. Paper presented at the Association for the Advancement of Behavior Therapy Annual Meeting, New Orleans, LA.

Pust, S., Mohnen, S. M., & Schneider, S. (2008). Individual and social environment influences on smoking in children and adolescents. *Public Health, 122*(12), 1324–1330.

Puzzanchera, C. M. (2003). Juvenile court placement of adjudicated youth, 1990–1999. *OJJDP Fact Sheet, 5*.

Ramsey, F., Ussery-Hall, A., Garcia, D., McDonald, G., Easton, A., Kambon, M., et al. (2008). Prevalence of selected risk behaviors and chronic diseases—behavioral risk factor surveillance system (BRFSS), 39 steps communities, United States, 2005. *MMWR Surveillance Summary, 57*(11), 1–20.

Reid, G. J., Irvine, J., McCrindle, B. W., Sananes, R., Ritvo, P. G., Siu, S. C., et al. (2004). Prevalence and correlates of successful transfer from pediatric to adult health care among a cohort of young adults with complex congenital heart defects. *Pediatrics, 113*, e197–e205.

Reid, G., McCrindle, B., Sananes, R., & Ritvo, P. (2004). Prevalence and correlates of successful transfer from pediatric to adult health care among a cohort of young adults with complex congenital heart defects. *Pediatrics, 113,* e197–e205.

Resnicow, K. (2002). Obesity prevention and treatment in youth: What is known? In F. L. Trowbridge & D. Kibbe (Eds.), *Childhood obesity: Partnerships for research and prevention* (pp. 11–30). Washington, DC: ILSI Press.

Resnicow, K. (2008, April). *Motivational interviewing: Applications to child health populations.* Paper presented at the Child Health Conference, Miami, FL.

Resnicow, K., Campbell, M. K., Carr, C., McCarty, F., Wang, T., Periasamy, S., et al. (2004). Body and soul. A dietary intervention conducted through African-American churches. *American Journal of Preventive Medicine, 27*(2), 97–105.

Resnicow, K., Davis, R., & Rollnick, S. (2006). Motivational interviewing for pediatric obesity: Conceptual issues and evidence review. *Journal of American Dietetic Assocociation, 106,* 2024–2033.

Resnicow, K., Jackson, A., Wang, T., Dudley, W., & Baranowski, T. (2001). A motivational interviewing intervention to increase fruit and vegetable intake through black churches: Results of the Eat for Life Trial. *American Journal of Public Health, 91,* 1686–1693.

Resnicow, K., & McMaster, F. (in press). Motivational interviewing: Moving from why to how with autonomy support. *International Journal of Behavioral Nutrition and Physical Activity.*

Resnicow, K., Taylor, R., & Baskin, M. (2005). Results of Go Girls: A nutrition and physical activity intervention for overweight African American adolescent females conducted through Black churches. *Obesity Research, 13*(10), 1739–1748.

Resnicow, K., Yaroch, A. L., Davis, A., Wang, D. T., Carter, S., Slaughter, L., et al. (2000). GO GIRLS!: Results from a nutrition and physical activity program for low-income, overweight African American adolescent females. *Health Education and Behavior, 27*(5), 616–631.

Reyna, V. F., & Farley, F. (2006). Risk and rationality in adolescent decision making: Implications for theory, practice, and public policy. *Psychological Science in the Public Interest, 7*(1), 1–44.

Rice, F. P. & Dolgin, K. G. (2008). *The adolescent: Development, relationships, and culture* (12th ed.). Boston: Pearson Education.

Rickman, R. L., Lodico, M., & DiClemente, R. J. (1994). Sexual communication is associated with condom use by sexually active incarcerated adolescents. *Journal of Adolescent Health, 15*(5), 383–388.

Rickwood, D. J., Deane, F. P., & Wison, C. J. (2007). When and how do young people seek professional help for mental health problems? *Medical Journal of Australia, 187,* S35–S39.

Roberts, M. E., Tchanturia, K., Stahl, D., Southgate, L., & Treasure, J. (2007). A systematic review and meta-analysis of set shifting ability in eating disorders. *Psychological Medicine, 37*(8), 1075–1084.

Rogers, C. R. (1959). A theory of therapy, personality, and interpersonal relationships as developed in the client-centered framework. In S. Koch (Ed.), *Psychology: The study of a science. Vol.3. Formulations of the person and the social contexts* (pp. 184–256). New York: McGraw-Hill.

Rollnick, S., Miller, W. R., & Butler, C. C. (2008). *Motivational interviewing in health care: Helping patients change behavior.* New York: Guilford Press.

Rosario, M., Hunter, J., Maguen, S., Gwadz, M., & Smith, R. (2001). The coming-out process and its adaptational and health-related associations among gay, lesbian, and bisexual youths: Stipulation and exploration of a model. *American Journal of Community Psychology, 29,* 133–160.

Rosengard, C., Stein, L. A. R., Barnett, N. P., Monti, P. M., Golembeske, C., Lebeau-Craven, R., et al. (2007). Randomized clinical trial of motivational enhancement of substance use treatment among incarcerated adolescents: Post-release condom non-use. *Journal of HIV/AIDS Prevention in Children and Youth, 8*(2), 45–64.

Rosengren, D. (in press). *Building motivational interviewing skills: A practitioner workbook.* New York: Guilford Press.

Rossler, W., Joachim Salize, H., Van Os, J., & Riecher-Rossler, A. (2005). Size of burden of schizophrenia and psychotic disorders. *European Neuropsychopharmacology, 15*(4), 399–409.

Rotgers, F., Morgenstern, J., & Walters, S. T. (2003). *Treating substance abuse: Theory and technique* (2nd ed.). New York: Guilford Press.

Rubak, S., Sandlbaek, A., Lauritzen, T., Borch-Johnsen, K., & Christensen, B. (2006). An education and training course in motivational interviewing influence: GP's professional behaviour. *British Journal of General Practice, 56*(527), 429–436.

Rudolf, M., Christie, D., McElhone, S., Sahota, P., Dixey, R., Walker, J., et al. (2006). WATCH IT: A community based programme for obese children and adolescents. *Archives of Disease in Childhood, 91,* 736–739.

Safe Schools Coalition of Washington. (1999). Eighty-three thousand youth: Selected findings of eight population-based studies as they pertain to anti-gay harassment and the safety and well-being of sexual minority students. Retrieved January 10, 2009, *www.safeschoolscoalition.org/theydonteven-knowme.pdf.*

Sanchez, F. (2001). *A values-based intervention for alcohol problems.* Unpublished doctoral dissertation, University of Mexico, Albuquerque.

Schmidt, U., Landau, S., Pombo-Carril, M., Bara-Carril, N., Reid, Y., Murray, K., et al. (2006). Does personalized feedback improve the outcome of cognitive-behavioural guided self-care in bulimia nervosa?: A preliminary randomized controlled trial. *British Journal of Clinical Psychology, 45*(1), 111–121.

Schmidt, U., Lee, S., Beecham, J., Perkins, S., Treasure, J., Yi, I., et al. (2007). A randomized controlled trial of family therapy and cognitive behavior therapy guided self-care for adolescents with bulimia nervosa and related disorders. *American Journal of Psychiatry, 164*(4), 591–598.

Schmidt, U., & Treasure, J. (2006). Anorexia nervosa: Valued and visible. A cognitive-interpersonal maintenance model and its implications for research and practice. *British Journal of Clinical Psychology, 45*(3), 343–366.

Schmiege, S. J., Broaddus, M. R., Levin, M., & Bryan, A. D. (2009). Randomized trial of group interventions to reduce HIV/STD risk and change theoretical mediators among detained adolescents. *Journal of Consulting and Clinical Psychology, 77*(1), 38–50.

Schoener, E. P., Madeja, C. L., Henderson, M. J., Ondersma, S. J., & Janisse, J. J. (2006). Effects of motivational interviewing training on mental health therapist behavior. *Drug and Alcohol Dependence, 89,* 269–275.

Schulenberg, J., Maggs, J. L., Steinman, K. J., & Zucker, R. A. (2001). Development matters: Taking the long view on substance abuse etiology and intervention during adolescence. In P. M. Monti, S. M. Colby, & T. A. O'Leary (Eds.), *Adolescents, alcohol, and substance abuse: Reaching teens through brief interventions* (pp. 19–57). New York: Guilford Press.

Schwartz, R. P., Hamre, R., Dietz, W. H., Wasserman, R. C., Slora, E. J., Myers, E. F., et al. (2007). Office-based motivational interviewing to prevent childhood obesity: a feasibility study. *Archives of Pediatrics and Adolescent Medicine, 161*(5), 495–501.

Schwarzer, R. & Luszczynsko, A. (2006). Self-efficacy, adolescents' risk taking behaviors, and health. In F. Pajares & T. Urdan (Eds.), *Self-efficacy beliefs of adolescents.* Charlotte, NC: Information Age.

Selvini, M. P., Boscolo, L., Cecchin, G., & Prata, G. (1980). Hypothesizing–circularity–neutrality: Three guidelines for the conductor of the session. *Family Process, 19,* 3–12.

Semple, S. J., Patterson, T. L., & Grant, I. (2004). Psychosocial characteristics and sexual risk behavior of HIV+ men who have anonymous sex partners. *Psychology and Health, 19,* 71–87.

Shechtman, Z. (2002). Child group psychotherapy in the school at the threshold of a new millennium. *Journal of Counseling and Development, 80,* 293–299.

Sepulveda, A. R., López, C., Todd, G., Whitaker, W., & Treasure, J. (2008). An examination of the impact of the Maudsley eating disorders collaborative care skills workshops on the wellbeing of carers: A pilot study. *Social Psychiatry and Psychiatric Epidemiology, 43*(7), 584–591.

Sepulveda, A. R., López, C. A., Macdonald, P., & Treasure, J. (2008). Feasibility and acceptability of DVD and telephone coaching-based skills training for carers of people with an eating disorder. *International journal of Eating Disorders, 41*(4), 318–325.

Shoptaw, S., Reback, C. J., Froshch, D. L., & Rawson, R. A. (1998). Stimulant abuse treatment as HIV prevention. *Journal of Addictive Diseases, 17,* 19–32.

Siegler, R. S. (1995). Children's thinking: How does change occur? In F. E. Weinert & W. Schnieder (Eds.), *Memory performance and competencies: Issues in growth and development* (pp. 405–430). Hillsdale, NJ: Erlbaum.

Simons-Morton, B., Crump, A. D., Haynie, D. L., Saylor, K. E., Eitel, P., & Yu, K. (1999). Psychosocial, school, and parent factors associated with recent smoking among early-adolescent boys and girls. *Preventive Medicine, 28*(2), 138–148.

Sindelar, H. A., Abrantes, A. M., Hart, C., Lewander, W., & Spirito, A. (2004). Motivational interviewing in pediatric practice. *Current Problems in Pediatric and Adolescent Health Care, 34*(9), 322–339.

Skiba, R., & Peterson, R. (1999). The dark side of zero tolerance: Can punishment lead to safe schools? *Phi Delta Kappan, 80,* 372–382.

Slavet, J. D., Stein, L. A. R., Klein, J. L., Colby, S. M., Barnett, N. P., & Monti, P. M. (2005). Piloting the family check-up with incarcerated adolescents and their parents. *Psychological Services, 2*(2), 122–132.

Smith, C. P., Firth, D., Bennett, S., Howard, C., & Chisolm, P.(1998). Ketoacidosis occurring in newly diagnosed and established diabetic children. *Acta Paediatrica Scandinavica, 87*(5), 537–541.

Smith, D. C. & Hall, J. A. (2007). Strengths-oriented referrals for teens (SORT): Giving balanced feedback to teens and families. *Health Social Work, 32*, 69–72.

Smith, D. C., Hall, J. A., Williams, J. K., An, H., & Gotman, N. (2006). Comparative efficacy of family and group treatment for adolescent substance abuse. *American Journal of Addictions, 15*(Suppl. 1), 131–136.

Spirito, A., Monti, P. M., Barrett, N. P., Colby, S. M., Sindelar, H., Rohsenow, D. J., et al. (2004). A randomized clinical trial of a brief motivational intervention for alcohol-positive adolescents treated in an emergency department. *Journal of Pediatrics, 145*, 396–402.

Spruijt-Metz, D. (1999). *Adolescence, affect and health*. London: Psychology Press.

Spruijt-Metz, D., Nguyen-Michel, S. T., Goran, M. I., Chou, C. P., & Huang, T. T. (2008). Reducing sedentary behavior in minority girls via a theory-based, tailored classroom media intervention. *International Journal of Pediatric Obesity, 3*(4), 240–248.

Spruijt-Metz, D., & Saelens, B. (2005). Behavioral aspects of physical activity in childhood and adolescence. In M. I. Goran & M. Southern (Eds.), *Handbook of pediatric obesity: Etiology, pathophysiology and prevention* (pp. 227–250). Boca Raton, FL: Taylor & Francis/CRC Press.

Stall, R., Duran, L., Wisniewski, S. R., Friedman, M. S., Marshal, M. P., McFarland, W., et al. (2009). Running in place: Implications of HIV incidence estimates among urban men who have sex with men in the United States and other industrialized countries. *AIDS and Behavior, 13*(4), 615–629.

Stearns, E., Moller, S., Blau, J., & Potochnick, S. (2007). Staying back and dropping out: The relationship between grade retention and school dropout. *Sociology of Education, 80*, 210–240.

Stein, L. A. R. (2004, December). *Preliminary findings of a randomized clinical trial in a juvenile correctional setting*. Paper presented at NIDA conference, Rockville, MD.

Stein, L. A. R., Colby, S. M., Barnett N. P., Monti, P. M., Golembeske, C., & Lebeau-Craven, R. (2006a). Validity of a brief alcohol expectancy questionnaire for adolescents: AEQ-AB. *Journal of Child and Adolescent Substance Abuse. 16*(2), 115–125.

Stein, L. A. R., Colby, S. M., Barnett, N. P., Monti, P. M., Golembeske, C., Lebeau-Craven, R., et al. (2006b). Enhancing substance abuse treatment engagement in incarcerated adolescents. *Psychological Services, 3*, 25–34.

Stein, L. A. R., & Lebeau-Craven, R. (2002). Motivational interviews & relapse prevention for DWI: A pilot study. *Journal of Drug Issues, 32*, 1051–1070.

Stein, L. A. R., Slavet, J., Gingras, M., & Golembeske, C. (2004). *Brief screening in juvenile detention using the Massachusetts Youth Screening Inventory–2*. Unpublished internal report, Brown University.

Steinberg, L. (1990). Autonomy, conflict, and harmony in the family relationship. In S. S. Feldman & G. L. Elliott (Eds.), *At the threshold: The developing adolescent* (pp. 255–276). Cambridge, MA: Harvard University Press.

Steinberg, L. (2005). *Adolescence* (7th ed.). Boston: McGraw-Hill.

Steinhausen, H.-C. (2002). The outcome of anorexia nervosa in the 20th century. *American Journal of Psychiatry, 159,* 1284–1293.

Steinhausen, H. C. (2009). Outcome of eating disorders. *Child and Adolescent Psychiatric Clinics of North America, 18*(1), 225–242.

Story, M. T., Neumark-Stzainer, D. R., Sherwood, N. E., Holt, K., Sofka, D., Trowbridge, F. L., et al. (2002). Management of child and adolescent obesity: Attitudes, barriers, skills, and training needs among health care professionals. *Pediatrics, 110*(1 Pt 2), 210–214.

Stott, N. C. H., Rollnick, S., & Pill, R. M. (1995). Innovation in clinical method: Diabetes care and negotiating skills. *Family Practice, 12*(4), 413–418.

Strauss, R. S., & Pollack, H. A. (2003). Social marginalization of overweight children. *Archives of Pediatrics and Adolescent Medicine, 157*(8), 746–752.

Striegel-Moore, R., DeBar, L., Wilson, G., Dickerson, J., Rosselli, F., Perrin, N., et al. (2007). Health services use in eating disorders. *Psychological Medicine, 2,* 1–10.

Suarez, M., & Mullins, S. (2008). Motivational interviewing and pediatric health behavior interventions. *Journal of Developmental Behavior Pediatrics, 29*(5), 417–428.

Substance Abuse and Mental Health Services Administration (SAMHSA). 2008. Results from the 2007 *National Survey on Drug Use and Health: National Findings* (Office of Applied Studies, DHHS Publication No. SMA 08-4343). Rockville, MD: Author.

Sue, S. (2008). Cultural competency: From philosophy to research and practice. *Journal of Community Psychology, 34*(2), 237–245.

Sussman, S. (2002). Effects of sixty six adolescent tobacco use cessation trials and seventeen prospective studies of self-initiated quitting. *Tobacco Induced Diseases, 1*(1), 35–81.

Sussman, S. (2005). Risk factors for and prevention of tobacco use. *Pediatric Blood and Cancer, 44*(7), 614–619.

Sussman, S., Dent, C. W., & Lichtman, K. L. (2001). Project EX: Outcomes of a teen smoking cessation program. *Addictive Behaviors, 26*(3), 425–438.

Sussman, S., Lichtman, K., Ritt, A., & Pallonen, U. E. (1999). Effects of thirty-four adolescent tobacco use cessation and prevention trials on regular users of tobacco products. *Substance Use and Misuse, 34*(11), 1469–1503.

Sussman, S., Sun, P., & Dent, C. W. (2006). A meta-analysis of teen cigarette smoking cessation. *Health Psychology, 25*(5),549–557.

Swan, M., Schwartz, S., Berg, B., Walker, D., Stephens, R., & Roffman, R. (2008). The teen marijuana check-up: An in-school protocol for eliciting voluntary self-assessment of marijuana use. *Journal of Social Work Practice in the Addictions, 8*(3), 284–302.

Swanson, A. J., Pantalon, M. V., & Cohen, K. R. (1999). Motivational interviewing and treatment adherence among psychiatrically and dually diagnosed patients. *Journal of Nervous and Mental Disease, 187,* 630–635.

Taveras, E. M., Berkey, C. S., Rifas-Shiman, S. L., Ludwig, D. S., Rockett, H. R.

H., Field, A. E., et al. (2005). Association of consumption of fried food away from home with body mass index and diet quality in older children and adolescents. *Pediatrics, 116*(4), e518–524.

Teplin, L. (2001). *Mental health: An emerging issue.* Atlanta, GA: Annual Conference of American Correctional Health Services Association.

Teplin, L. A., Abram, K. M., McClelland, G. M., Dulan, M. K., & Mericle, A. A. (2002). Psychiatric disorders in youth in juvenile detention. *Archives of General Psychology, 59*, 1133–1143.

Teplin, L. A., Mericle, A. A., McClelland, G. M., & Abram, K. M. (2003). HIV and AIDS risk behaviors in juvenile detainees: Implications for public health policy. *American Journal of Public Health, 93*, 906–912.

Thornberry, T. P., Tolnay, S. E., Flanagan, T. J., & Glynn, P. (1991). Children in custody 1987: A comparison of public and private juvenile custody facilities. Washington, DC: Office of Juvenile Justice and Delinquency Prevention.

Tiggemann, M., & Anesbury, T. (2000). Negative stereotyping of obesity in children: The role of controllability beliefs. *Journal of Applied Social Psychology, 30*(9), 1977–1993.

Titus, J. C., Dennis, M. L., Diamond, G., Godley, S. H., Babor, T., Donaldson, J., et al. (1999). *Treatment of adolescent marijuana abuse: A randomized clinical trial. Presentation 1: Structure of the Cannabis Youth Treatment Study.*

Tober, G., Godfrey, C., Parrott, S., Copello, A., Farrin, A., Hodgson, R., et al. (2005). Setting standards for training and competence: The UK alcohol treatment trial. *Alcohol and Alcoholism, 40*, 413–418.

Tobler, N. S. (2000). Lessons learned. *Journal of Primary Prevention, 20*(4), 261–274.

Tobler, N. S., & Stratton, H. H. (1997). Effectiveness of school-based drug prevention programs: A meta-analysis of the research. *Journal of Primary Prevention, 18*, 71–128.

Treasure, J. (2007). Getting beneath the phenotype of anorexia nervosa: the search for viable endophenotypes and genotypes. *Canadian Journal of Psychiatry, 52*(4), 212–209.

Treasure, J., Katzman, M., Schmidt, U., Troop, N., Todd, G., & de Silva, P. (1999). Engagement and outcome in the treatment of bulimia nervosa: first phase of a sequential design comparing motivation enhancement therapy and cognitive behavioural therapy. *Behaviour, Research and Therapy, 37*(5), 405–418.

Treasure, J., Murphy, T., Szmukler, G., Tood, G., Gavan, K., & Joyce, J. (2001). The experience of caregiving for severe mental illness: a comparison between anorexia nervosa and psychosis. *Social Psychiatry and Psychiatric Epidemiology, 36*(7), 343–347.

Treasure, J., & Schmidt, U. (2008). Motivational interviewing in eating disorders. In H. Arkowitz, H. A. Westra, W. R. Miller, & S. Rollnick (Eds.), *Motivational interviewing in the treatment of psychological problems* (pp. 194–224). New York: Guilford Press.

Treasure, J., Sepulveda, A., MacDonald, P., Whitaker, P., López, C., Zabala, M, et al. (2008). Interpersonal maintaining factors in eating disorder: Skill sharing interventions for carers. *International Journal of Child and Adolescent Health, 1*(4), 331–338.

Treasure, J., Sepulveda, A. R., Whitaker, W., Todd, G., López, C., & Whitney,

J. (2007). Collaborative care between professionals and non-professionals in the management of eating disorders: A description of workshops focused on interpersonal maintaining factors. *European Eating Disorders Review, 15,* 15–24.

Treasure, J., Smith, G. D., & Crane, A. M. (2007). *Skills-based learning for caring for a loved one with an eating disorder.* Hampshire, UK: Routledge/Taylor & Francis.

Treasure, J., Tchanturia, K., & Schmidt, S. (2005). Developing a model of the treatment for eating disorder: using neuroscience research to examine the how rather than the what of change. *Counselling and Psychotherapy Research, 5,* 187–190.

Treasure, J. L., & Ward, A. (1997). A practical guide to the use of motivational interviewing in anorexia nervosa. *European Eating Disorders Review, 5,* 102–114.

Treasure, J., Whitaker, W., Whitney, J., & Schmidt, U. (2005). Working with families of adults with anorexia nervosa. *Journal of Family Therapy, 27,* 158–170.

Trepper, T. (1991). Senior editor's comments. In M. Worden, *Adolescents and their families: An introduction to assessment and intervention.* New York: Haworth Press.

Troiano, R. P., Berrigan, D., Dodd, K. W., Masse, L. C., Tilert, T., & McDowell, M. (2008). Physical activity in the United States measured by accelerometer. *Medicine and Science in Sports and Exercise, 40*(1), 181–188.

Vallerand, R. J. (1997). Toward a hierarchial model of intrinsic and extrinsic motivation. In Z. M. Zanna (Ed.), *Advances in experimental social psychology* (pp. 271–360). New York: Academic Press.

van den Bree, M. B. M., & Pickworth, W. B. (2005). Risk factors predicting changes in marijuana involvement in teenagers. *Archives of General Psychiatry, 62,* 311–319.

Vaughn, M. G., & Howard, M. O. (2004). Adolescent substance abuse treatment: A synthesis of controlled evaluations. *Research on Social Work Practice, 14*(5), 325–335.

Wade, T. D., Frayne, A., Edwards, S., Robertson, T., & Gilchrist, P. (2009). Motivational change in an inpatient anorexia nervosa population and implications for treatment. *Australian and New Zealand Journal of Psychiatry, 43*(3), 235–243.

Wagner, E. F. & Austin, A. M. (2009). Problem solving and social skills training. In D. Springer & A. Rubin (Eds.), *Substance abuse treatment for youths and adults, clinician's guide to evidence-based practice series.* Hoboken, NJ: Wiley.

Wagner, E., & Macgowan, M. (2006). School-based group treatment for adolescent substance abuse. In H. A. Liddle & C. L. Rowe (Eds.), *Adolescent substance abuse: Research and clinical advances* (pp. 333–356). New York: Cambridge University Press.

Waldron, H. B., Slesnick, N., Brody, J. L., Turner, C. W., & Peterson, T. R. (2001). Treatment outcomes for adolescent substance abuse at 4- and 7-month assessments. *Journal of Consulting and Clinical Psychology, 69,* 802–813.

Waldron, H. B., & Turner, C. W. (2008). Evidence-based psychosocial treatments for adolescent substance abuse. *Journal of Clinical Child and Adolescent Psychology, 37*(1), 238–261.

Walker, D. D., Roffman, R. A., Stephens, R. S., Berghuis, J., & Kim, W. (2006). Motivational enhancement therapy for adolescent marijuana users: A preliminary randomized controlled trial. *Journal of Consulting and Clinical Psychology, 74*(3), 628–632.

Walters, S. T., Vader, A. M., Harris, T. R., Field, C. A., & Jouriles, E. N. (2009). Dismantling motivational interviewing and feedback for college drinkers: A randomized clinical trial. *Journal of Consulting and Clinical Psychology, 77*(1), 64–73.

Wang, M. Q., Fitzhugh, E. C., Lee, G. B., Turner, L. W., Eddy, J. M., & Westerfield, R. C. (1998). Prospective social-psychological factors of adolescent smoking progression. *Journal of Adolescent Health, 24*(1), 2–9.

Weigensberg, M. J., Lane, C. J., Winners, O., Wright, T., Nguyen-Rodriguez, S., Goran, M. I., et al. (2009). Acute effects of stress-reduction Interactive Guided Imagery(SM) on salivary cortisol in overweight Latino adolescents. *Journal of Alternative and Complementary Medicine, 15*(3), 297–303.

Weinstein, A. G., & Faust, D. (1997). Maintaining theophylline compliance/adherence in severely asthmatic children: The role of psychologic functioning of the child and family. *Annals of Allergy, Asthma, and Immunology, 79*, 311–318.

Weiss Weiwel, E. (2009, February 17). *HIV/AIDS surveillance and epidemiology in New York City.* Presentation delivered at the annual meeting of the New York City Department of Health and Mental Hygiene Planning and Prevention Group, New York.

Weist, M. D., Evans, S. W., & Lever, N. A. (Eds.). (2003). *Handbook of school mental health: Advancing practice and research.* New York: Springer.

Werner, M. J. (1995). Principles of brief intervention for adolescent alcohol, tobacco, and other drug use. *Substance Abuse, 42*, 335–349.

Westra, H. A. (2004). Managing resistance in cognitive behavioural therapy: The application of motivational interviewing in mixed anxiety and depression. *Cognitive Behavior Therapy, 33*, 161–175.

Westra, H. A., Arkowitz, H., & Dozois, D. J. (2008, November). *Motivational interviewing as a pretreatment to CBT for generalized anxiety disorder: Results of a randomized controlled trial.* Paper presented at the annual meeting of the Association for Behavioral and Cognitive Therapies, Orlando, FL.

Whitney, J., & Eisler, I. (2005). Theoretical and empirical models around caring for someone with an eating disorder: The reorganization of family life and inter-personal maintenance factors. *Journal of Mental Health, 14*(6), 575–585.

Whitney, J., Haigh, R., Weinman, J., & Treasure, J. (2007). Caring for people with eating disorders: Factors associated with psychological distress and negative caregiving appraisals in carers of people with eating disorders. *British Journal of Clinical Psychology, 46*(4), 413–428.

WHO. (1997). *Obesity: Preventing and managing the global epidemic. Report of a WHO Consultation on Obesity.* Geneva: WHO.

WHO. (2001). *The WHO World Health Report: New understanding, new hope.* Geneva: Author.

WHO. (2005). Obesity and overweight. Retrieved May 18, 2009, 2009, from *www.who.int/mediacentre/factsheets/fs311/en/index.html.*

Williams, G. C. (2002). Improving patients' health through supporting the autonomy of patients and providers. In E. L. Deci & R. M. Ryan (Eds.), *Handbook of self-determination research* (p. 233–254). Rochester, NY: University of Rochester Press.

Williams, G. C., Cox, E. M. Kouides, R., & Deci, E. L. (1999). Presenting the facts about smoking to adolescents. *Archives of Pediatric and Adolescent Medicine, 153,* 959–964.

Winickoff, J. P., Hillis, V. J., Palfrey, J. S., Perrin, J. M., & Rigotti, N. A. (2003). A smoking cessation intervention for parents of children who are hospitalized for respiratory illness: The stop tobacco outreach program. *Pediatrics, 111,* 140–145.

Winters, K. C., & Leitten, W. (2007). Brief intervention for drug-abusing adolescents in a school setting. *Psychology of Addictive Behaviors, 21*(2), 249–254.

Wolfenden, L., Campbell, E., Walsh, R., Raoul, A., & Wiggers, J. (2003). Smoking cessation interventions for in-patients: A selective review with recommendations for hospital-based health professionals. *Drug and Alcohol Review, 22*(4), 437–452.

Wood, V. D., & Shoroye, A. (1993). Sexually transmitted disease among adolescents in the juvenile justice system of the District of Columbia. *Journal of the National Medical Association, 85*(6), 435–439.

Woodall, W. G., Delaney, H. D., Kunitz, S. J., Westerberg, V. S., & Zhao, H. (2007). A randomized trial of a DWI intervention program for first offenders: Intervention outcomes and interactions with antisocial personality disorder among a primarily American-Indian Sample. *Alcohol Clinical Experimental Research, 31*(6), 974–987.

Woodruff, S. I., Edwards, C. C., Conway, T. L., & Elliott, S. P. (2001). Pilot Test of an Internet virtual world chat room for rural teen smokers. *Journal of Adolescent Health, 29,* 239–243.

Wysocki, T., Taylor, A., Hough, B. S., Linscheid, T. R., Yeates, K. O., & Naglieri, J. A. (1996). Deviation from developmentally appropriate self-care autonomy: Association with diabetes outcome. *Diabetes Care, 19,* 119–125.

Yan, A. F., Chiu, Y.-W., Stoesen, C. A., & Wang, M. Q. (2007). STD-/HIV-related sexual risk behaviors and substance use among U.S. rural adolescents. *Journal of the National Medical Association, 99,* 1386–1394.

Young, D. W., Dembo, R., & Henderson, C. E. (2007). A national survey of substance abuse treatment for juvenile offenders. *Journal of Substance Abuse Treatment, 32,* 255–266.

Zimmer-Gembeck, M. J., & Helfand, M. (2008). Ten years of longitudinal research on U.S. adolescent sexual behavior: Developmental correlates of sexual intercourse, and the importance of age, gender and ethnic background. *Developmental Review, 153*–224.

Index

Page numbers followed by *f* indicate figure, *t* indicate table